HEAR
THE BEAT,
FEEL THE
MUSIC

HEAR THE BEAT, *FEEL* THE MUSIC

COUNT, CLAP AND TAP YOUR WAY
TO REMARKABLE RHYTHM

JAMES JOSEPH

VIDEO ALERT: This book requires the internet to view free instructional videos at **HearTheBeatFeelTheMusic.com**. *Disclaimer:* Due to copyright law, some music may only be viewable in the United States.

BlueChip Publishers
Jackson Hole, Wyoming

This book requires you to use the internet to view free instructional videos at HearTheBeatFeelTheMusic.com. The videos are hosted on YouTube. If, due to copyright law, YouTube blocks a video, every effort will be made by the author to find a replacement. Also, due to copyright law, which varies from country to country, some music may only be viewable in the United States.

Printed in the United States of America.

Cover and interior design by 1106 Design.

ISBN 978-0-930251-48-2
Kindle (Mobi) ISBN 978-0-930251-50-5
EPUB ISBN 978-0-930251-51-2
PDF ISBN 978-0-930251-49-9

Library of Congress Control Number: 2017912663

BlueChip Publishers
Jackson Hole, Wyoming
BlueChipPublishers.com

Available for purchase in bulk and in custom editions.

Contact the author at jim@ihatetodance.com
Visit the author's websites at HearTheBeatFeelTheMusic.com and iHateToDance.com

First Edition, Version 1.0

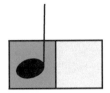

Acknowledgments

I'm indebted to dance educator Skippy Blair (swingworld.com) for her support and guidance. I also want to thank Skippy and her organization, the Golden State Dance Teachers Association (GSDTA), for letting me use some of their terms and concepts (credited throughout the book). Skippy did not read the final manuscript of the book and she did not approve or disapprove of what I have written.

A big thanks to Amy Daniels, who has been by my side, in the trenches, as I wrote this book. She was my sounding board, my technical editor and my search-and-rescue team.

Thanks to Sarah Grusmark, Senior Adjunct Professor, ULV, and Yvonne Belin for reading the manuscript. Thanks to my editors, Danielle Adams and Charlie Wilson. Thanks to my advisors Carl Schreier and Bill and Diane Tjenos. Thanks to my publishing maven, Ina Stern. And a special thanks to Agent Natasha.

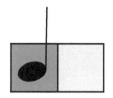

Contents

Music can change the world because it can change people.

— BONO

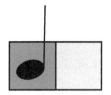

Introduction

YOU LOVE MUSIC...SURE.

And you may even know a lot about it. Or you may know nothing—it doesn't matter. This book isn't about *knowing* music in your head, it's about connecting to it at a deeper level. It's about *feeling* it in your bones. It's about creating a rhythmic connection.

But this word "rhythm" bugs me. It's used in different ways and I don't always know what people mean. So let me spell out what you'll get from this book:

1. You'll learn how to hear the beat of music. You'll learn about *sets of 8*, also known as the *8-count*, which are the key to hearing the beat. You'll learn how to count the sets of 8, because that's how you rhythmically train your ear.

2. You'll learn how to clap. This will help you connect to music, because clapping is like being an instrument in the band. Of course, this will also help when

you're sitting in an audience and the crowd begins to clap. Audiences are often pretty bad at clapping, which I get into in Chapter 3.

3. You'll learn how to identify the structure of music. This is known as *phrasing.* This will start you on the path to better *musicality,* because it'll help you to predict where the music is going. It'll give you the somewhat useless skill of being able to predict and punch the air to a big accent or hit in the music (but I bet your friends will find that cool). There's more: according to the field of *biomusicology,* the study of biology and music, if you can predict where the music is going, you'll enjoy it more. Yup, lying on the couch and chilling to music is about to get better.

And if you think you're "rhythmically challenged"—that is, you think you can't hear the beat, which might be better described as "beat challenged"—boy, have I got some good news. *Being rhythmically challenged is not a lack of ability; it's a lack of education.* As a kid, were you taught how to hear the beat? I think not.

MUSICIAN VERSUS DANCER ALERT: You could learn the beat and phrasing from a musician, but a musician will teach you *music theory,* which is complicated and TMI (too much information). The method in this book is used by dance choreographers; it's related to music theory, but it's easier and better suited to non-musicians. *If you're a musician, please don't have a heart attack when you read this book.* Just be aware that musicians deal with music in a different way than dancers, which I talk about in Chapter 1. Note that terms I use that musicians also use may differ in meaning, so watch for LINGO ALERTS, which will tip you off to confusing language.

GIVE ME FEEDBACK: I have no talent in music. When I struggle with things, like how to hear the beat, I like to figure out an easy way to do it. Then I like to share it and, hopefully, make it a fun read. If you think I'm wrong about something, please let me know. If an explanation is not clear, give me a holler. If you've got a gripe, throw me an email (jim@ihatetodance.com). I'm always looking for a better way.

Using This Book

This book uses music on YouTube because you can listen to popular music, ahem, on the cheap (a DVD or digital download, because of the licensing fees, would blow a hole in your wallet). *So you need an internet connection to watch videos.* Here's how things work:

- The link in this book to the videos is not a link to YouTube, it's a link to the web page for the book, HearTheBeatFeelTheMusic.com. Say what? No sweat, really. This web page has the video playlist, which is a list of all the YouTube videos that go with the book, laid out by chapter. The video playlist will make handling the book and YouTube easier.

- The videos are numbered by chapter. For example, "video 1.1" is the first video for Chapter 1; "video 1.2" is the second video for Chapter 1. If I say to watch the "video *series* 2.1," that means there will be more than one video and you need to scroll through them. In the video series 2.1, the first video is numbered 2.1.1, the second video is 2.1.2, etc.

- If I want you to click to a section in a video, I'll say something like, "Listen to the section from 1:15 to 1:45 minutes." That means listen from the one minute and 15 second mark to the one minute and 45 second mark. (*Note:* times could be off by a second or two.) It's easy to jump around a YouTube video by clicking anywhere in the progress bar.

- Over time, I may add videos or I may have to replace a video. *So don't be shocked if the book talks about a video but there's a replacement on the website.* If I do that, there will be an explanation in the blurb for the new video at HearTheBeatFeelTheMusic.com. COPYRIGHT ALERT: If YouTube blocks a video in your country because of copyright law, please let me know and I'll find a solution.

So, you ask yourself, *Can't anyone watch the videos for free on YouTube?* Yes, and in that sense, the web page for the book is a "free online course." So, you wonder, *Why shell out lunch money to buy this book?* Well, if you have some aptitude in music, the web page may be all you need. For the rest of us, mere mortals with no musical chops, I think you'll find this book—with explanations, exercises, motivational words and handholding—to be the fastest path to achieving remarkable rhythm.

POPULAR MUSIC ALERT: I've chosen popular music because not only is it more fun to listen to, but popular music will show you that the music structures you're about to learn are very common. I use the phrase "popular music" loosely. I'm writing for an American audience and I'm talking about contemporary, mainstream, Western music. While there are millions of songs and everyone's taste in listening differs, my guess is that this book covers a lot of what you hear every day. For many of you, it probably covers most of what you hear. It also covers many genres of music, even if a particular song in that genre is not popular. So, in that sense, it also covers a lot of unpopular music. It does not refer to just the genre of "pop music," although pop music is popular music.

My Struggle to Hear the Beat

I know, you've listened to music your whole life so you're an expert, and you can name every Rolling Stones album and you have 57,000 tunes on your iDevice to prove it.

But if I played you 10 songs and asked you to tap your foot to the beat with 100 percent confidence, I bet you wouldn't be so sure and you'd have to guess. You may be correct, but you'd be guessing.

When I was learning to partner dance I guessed a lot. Sometimes I was right, probably by chance (think: even a broken clock is right twice a day). And sometimes I was wrong. But I had polite partners who had the courtesy to *not* tell me that I was off the beat and to *not* tell me that my dancing sucked. All this gave me the illusion that I had rhythm. So I was not only rhythmically challenged but I didn't know it. Occasionally, a partner would tell me I was off the beat, and I'd think she was nuts. So I was also in denial.

I finally realized I had a problem and sought help. Naturally, I asked people who were good at music—people with talent. They all made it seem so easy: "It's in the music, just feel it." I felt nothing. I'd go in and out of periods of thinking that it took talent to hear the beat.

Fortunately, I took some workshops with Swing Dance Hall of Famer Skippy Blair (swingworld.com). She taught me about the 8-count and phrasing in music, something I had not found anywhere else. I blossomed. While I still didn't have talent, I came to realize that what Skippy said was true: it was a lack of education and training that was holding me back.

One of the dances I was trying to learn was the Lindy Hop, the original swing dance, so I started collecting swing music, a type of jazz. I came across one song and had a breakthrough. It was the first song where I could hear the structure—the phrasing. I could hear not only the sets of 8 in the music, but also how the sets of 8 came together to form the bigger structure. I played this song over and over and I marveled at what I was hearing. For a brief period of time (very brief!) I felt like a genius. The song is "Gotta Do Some War Work, Baby" by Cootie Williams (1911–1985), a jazz trumpet player. We'll get into it in Chapter 1 and maybe things will click for you, too.

While this song gave me a foothold, the floodgates did not open. I was still befuddled by the vast majority of music. But I knew I was on to something and I was enjoying it. For two years I counted the sets of 8 obsessively, anytime and anywhere I heard music. Finally, it became natural and I stopped thinking about it. Finally, I could feel the beat. (No doubt, with a coach or guide like this book, I would have done it more quickly.)

Now I'm almost a virtuoso when it comes to tapping my foot and clapping my hands. I can even dance and, on a good night, not embarrass myself. Best of all, I enjoy listening to music more. At times, I even feel like I'm part of the band.

And that's my hope for you: that you find your groove and become that person who's "got rhythm."

Life is about rhythm. We vibrate, our hearts are pumping blood, we are a rhythm machine, that's what we are.

— MICKEY HART, DRUMMER FOR THE GRATEFUL DEAD

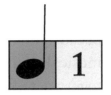

Count the Music

A LOT OF BRAINS out there will shut down at the thought of counting music. I beg, give it a try. It's just counting, not math. You'll only be counting to **8** and it's kind of fun, really.

Even if you can't hear the structure, music has structure. For non-musicians, the most important structural element to know is a *set of 8*, also known as an *8-count* and an eight-beat *mini-phrase*. If you can count the sets of 8, you've found the *underlying beat*.

A **set of 8** is a rhythmic grouping of eight beats, which defines the beat of the music (that's for 4/4 time music, which is explained in Chapter 4). In popular music, sets of 8 often repeat throughout a song, kind of the same way that sentences repeat in a piece of writing.

Also, like a sentence, a set of 8 usually has a theme. You need to listen for themes, because generally these themes are related to the musical count and the structure. To get you started on musical themes, I'll point them out as we listen to music in the next section of this chapter.

There's one other structural element, a *major phrase* (not to be confused with a *mini-phrase*), which I'll mention now because it'll help you hear the sets of 8. Essentially, the musical themes of the sets of 8 (mini-phrases) can come together to form a bigger theme, which is a *major phrase.* So major phrases, like paragraphs in a piece of writing, are part of the bigger structure in a piece of music. Hang tight, you'll hear two examples of this in a moment. Then we'll get further into major phrases in Chapter 6, "Phrasing."

On your journey to connect to the beat, pay attention to the drums. While music is made up of vocals, melody, harmony and drums, *it's the drums that create the underlying beat of music.* The drums and other percussion instruments are called the *percussion section* of the band. When you add the keyboard and guitars to the percussion section, it's often called the *rhythm section,* although the components of a rhythm section can vary from band to band.

Don't be fooled: sometimes the underlying beat sounds like it's coming from the vocals or melody. That's because the vocals and melody can be rhythmically aligned with the sets of 8. Knowing what to listen for can be tricky and I don't expect you, with an untrained ear, to always identify the rhythm section. But over time, you'll gain a sense for it. For now, just remember that the drums and percussion have the final word in establishing the beat, because that'll come in handy when you're up against difficult music.

LINGO ALERT: In my experience, "set of 8" and "8-count" are not terms that musicians use. If a musician wants to refer to a set of 8, they usually just call it a "phrase" of music. But musicians also use the word "phrase" to label other groupings of beats, so you may need clarification. That's why I like to use the term *mini-phrase* (a term coined by dance educator Skippy Blair) when talking about a set of 8. While *set of 8* and *mini-phrase* can be used synonymously, there's a little more to it. Mini-phrases can vary in length, which is why I referred to it above as an "eight-beat mini-phrase." As you'll see in Chapter 4, a mini-phrase in the waltz is six beats, which you can also call a *set of 6*.

Feel the Music

> *Don't count, feel! The only count I know, is Count Basie!*
> — Dawn Hampton, born 1928, performed at the Apollo Theater and the Savoy Ballroom

We'll get to counting music in a moment. First, it'll help to get a feel for the music; that is, to get a sense for hearing the sets of 8 without counting, because ultimately that's your endgame. There's more on how to do this later in the chapter. For now, let the next two songs wash over you and prime your brain for what's to come. Listen a few times and let your subconscious soak it in.

The first cut is the chorus from the song "Brother Louie," a number-one hit in the 1970s by the band Stories (original version by Hot Chocolate). While the whole song is an example of the bigger structure I want you to get familiar with (four sets of 8), I want to focus on just the chorus because the structure is so easy to hear. Go to HearTheBeatFeelTheMusic.com and watch **video 1.1**.

The chorus runs from 0:57 seconds to 1:15. As you listen, think about the structure in terms of four sets of 8 coming together, thematically, to create a major phrase of music. Here are the vocals for the four sets of 8 in the chorus of "Brother Louie":

1st set of 8:	*Louie Louie Louie Louieeeeeeeee*
2nd set of 8:	*Louie Louie Louie Louiiiiiiiiiiiiiiiiiiii*
3rd set of 8:	*Louie Louie Louie Louieeeeeeeee*
4th set of 8:	*Louie Louie you're gonna cryyyyy*

As you listen try to hear how a phrase of words aligns with a set of 8 in the music. Notice how a set of 8 stands out. Specifically, notice how, thematically, the first three sets of 8 set up something, which gets resolved in the fourth set of 8.

Ponder this concept of themes in music, and *setup and resolution* in particular, because they happen a lot. While *resolution* is more complicated than this, for now think of the music building up tension that gets released through the resolution. A resolution brings a sense of comfort or closure.

I chose the chorus of this song because it's drop-dead easy music, but most music will not be this easy. One reason it's easy is because the words line up with each set of 8 in the music. In harder music that's not always the case (I repeat:

vocals do not always line up with the sets of 8). If you have trouble or want to check your work, I count the sets of 8 in the chorus of this song in **video 1.5**, "Hear Sets of 8–Feel the Music." It's the first song.

Next, listen to a piece of old jazz, "Gotta Do Some War Work, Baby" by Cootie Williams. I hesitated to include this song because it's a harder song. But I think it's educational because it's a good example of musical themes. Plus, you've got to love the name *Cootie*.

This was my breakthrough piece of music, as I mentioned in the Introduction to the book. This is the song that opened the door for me and I hope it works for you. This was the first song where I could hear the thematic nature of a set of 8. It was this song that made me realize that I could become more rhythmic. If it doesn't click with you now, come back to it after you read Chapter 6.

Go to **video 1.2** on the website and listen to "Gotta Do Some War Work, Baby." Focus on the beginning of the song, the first 1:05 minutes, which have no vocals. There are five major phrases and each one runs for about 13 seconds.

In the first 1:05 minutes of the song the melody is prominent (in "Brother Louie" the vocals were prominent). While the tempo is fast and the beat isn't that pronounced, the melody, which lines up with the sets of 8, is in your face. But, in general, don't fall in love with melody because, like vocals, the melody of a song does not always line up with the sets of 8.

Listening to just the melody, notice how something builds up in the first three sets of 8 and then resolves in the fourth set of 8. This creates, thematically, a major phrase of music. This structure (four sets of 8) repeats throughout the song. The beauty of this song is that the melody and structure are aligned and very obvious. This structure of four sets of 8 is common in a lot of music, although typically it's not this easy to hear.

If you have trouble or want to check your work, I count the sets of 8 in this song in **video 1.5** (the second song).

These two songs were easy because the vocals or melody helped you to identify the sets of 8. But remember, while vocals and melody might sometimes be aligned with the sets of 8, they frequently are not. So, regardless of what you read on the internet, don't rely completely on vocals and melody.

Most music will be more difficult than the two examples above. In some music, sets of 8 may be darn near impossible to hear. But they're probably there—they're just "in" the music—and you'll be able to feel the **8s** even if you can't actually hear the **8s**. The way to develop this skill is by counting—counting the **8s**! Counting not only connects you to the music but it's a way to confirm that you've found the beat.

Some of you may already be familiar with sets of 8 but didn't know it. You might think, *Well, of course, I can feel the sets of 8 in music all the time.* Exactly! If this describes you, you should pick up counting very quickly.

Intro to Counting

To get started counting, watch the next video, which shows the relationship between the dancer's count and the musician's count. It's a good introduction to sets of 8 and it will answer that nagging question: How is it that sets of 8 define the beat of music?

Go to the website and watch **video 1.3**, "Intro to Sets of 8–How to Count Music." I'll wait...

The video you just watched showed how two four-beat **measures** are rhythmically paired to create a set of 8. The takeaway is this: while musicians count in four-beat measures (also called *bars*), dancers and non-musicians count in sets of 8. *You can translate the musician's count into the dancer's count by recognizing that* **count 1** *of the second measure is the same as* **count 5** *in a set of 8.* It looks like this:

1 2 3 4   5 6 7 8 – dancer's count (a *set of 8* or an *8-count*)
1 2 3 4   1 2 3 4 – musician's count (two four-beat *measures*)

Now that you know the theory behind sets of 8, you're ready for the next step: finding a **count 1** and counting.

ANOTHER MUSICIAN VERSUS DANCER ALERT: Sets of 8 are a dancer thing. They're better for identifying the structure in popular music, which you need for choreographing movement, a moot point to a musician. Sets of 8 are better for predicting where the music is going, whether you're a dancer or just a person who enjoys listening to music. Most importantly, sets of 8 and four-beat measures can coexist. For example, a bandleader often starts a band playing by saying, "One, two, three, four." Yet a dance teacher would start a class dancing (after the music has started) to the exact same song by saying, "Five, six, seven, eight."

Counting Sets of 8

Hearing sets of 8 is not a clear or logical process. It's not a science and there's not a right way to do it. I'll give you a place to start, some things to listen for. In the end, when you're good at it, you may not know how you do it. You might even be like one of those annoying people with talent who say, "It's in the music, just feel it."

The way to get started counting is simple: jump in and make mistakes!

You can jump into the music anywhere you like because sets of 8 usually repeat throughout a song. In fact, you may have to let a few sets of 8 go by before you can hear a **count 1** coming. When you think you hear the beat and a **count 1**, jump in and count to eight over and over: *one, two, three, four, five, six, seven, eight,* **one,** *two, three*…and so on. As you count, you'll wonder if you're counting correctly. There will be failed attempts. So stop and start over. It will be trial and error. This is how you train your ear.

(This may help or this may confuse you, but what the heck: Keep in mind that a set of 8 is a pretty short chunk of music. A set of 8 is only eight beats. So, when you listen to a song, a new set of 8 starts every few seconds. For example, if the tempo of a song is 60 beats per minute, which is slow, a new set of 8 will start every eight seconds. Most music will be faster than 60 beats per minute. That means that most sets of 8 will be less than eight seconds in length.)

To hear the sets of 8 you need to train your brain to listen for detail. You need to listen *actively* to all the different elements of the music. In particular, you need to listen for "clues" that reveal the structure. To keep it simple, I'll put the "clues" into two broad categories: listen for an accent or emphasis on **count 1**; and listen for a mini-phrase (set of 8) of music. Let's dig into these and see if you can get the hang of it:

1) *Listen for an accent or emphasis on* **count 1**. In addition to an accent or emphasis on **count 1**, also listen for an accent or emphasis on **count 5**, but to a lesser degree. **Counts 1** and **5** are the first beat of each measure. Often, but not always—I repeat, not always—those beats will sound stronger or sound different, especially **count 1**. Listening for an accent or emphasis on **count 1** is often an easy place to start because it's a specific beat of music.

But what's an "emphasis"?

Sometimes **count 1** is louder or has more strength or has more oomph. I'm calling that an *accent*. But sometimes **count 1** is not louder. Sometimes it has a manner or presence that's just different. I'm calling that an *emphasis*. It could be a heaviness or an emptiness. It could be some sort of transition point. Often what you hear on **count 1** is something you can't explain. I often don't know why **count 1** sounds different. Fortunately, it doesn't matter why, it only matters that you hear something different. In that way, try to develop a sense for "something" on **count 1**, not an intellect for it. Music will whiz by and there's no time to dissect it.

A good example of what I mean by an accent on **count 1** is the instrumental opening of "Hotel California" by the Eagles. But I decided not to link to it because YouTube is blocking a lot of the versions. If you find the song on your own, just listen to the first 50 seconds, which is two major phrases. Each major phrase runs for about 25 seconds. Note that there are accents on both the **count 1s** and the **count 5s** at about the same intensity, which I talk about in the next TIP.

MUSIC NOTE: Instead of "Hotel California," I've gone back to the first song I had chosen to show what I mean by an accent, "Dark Love." After I made the video with "Dark Love" (video 1.5) I learned that there's something tricky about the song. But I decided to turn this issue into a teachable moment because I like the song and I already made the video. At this point, the issue isn't important but I discuss it at the end of Chapter 4 under another MUSIC NOTE (*spoiler alert*: it has to do with time signature).

Go to the website and watch **video 1.4**, "Dark Love" by Robin Rogers. Note that the accents are not strong. The accents on the **count 1s** are soft and the accents on the

count 5s are even softer. You may question whether they're accented. That's good because I want you to have to think about it. I want you to get a feel for a lighter accent, which is common in music.

The first 32 beats (four sets of 8), which run from about 0:02 to 0:30 seconds, are instrumental (no vocals). Then the vocals kick in and the next 32 beats run from about 0:31 to 0:59 seconds. Note how her voice now accents the **count 1s** and the **count 5s**. (Ignore the two-beat "pickup" in the first two seconds of the song, before the first set of 8 starts.)

Jump in and try to count the sets of 8. If you have trouble or want to check your work, I count the sets of 8 in this song in **video 1.5** (the third song).

TIP: It's natural to hear *four-beat measures* because, like sets of 8, measures are "in" the music. I don't know if this will happen to you, but in my early years of training I went through a period where I could hear the four-beat measures but I couldn't hear the sets of 8. To my ear, it seemed like all the **count 5s** had accents as strong as the **count 1s**. I couldn't distinguish between the **1s** and the **5s**. I couldn't hear how measures were paired. If this happens to you, let a few more sets of 8 go by, especially the beginning of a new major phrase, which should give you a strong beginning point (see the next TIP). Also, try to hear how a four-beat measure, even though it has some integrity, often sounds incomplete, like half a sentence. If it sounds incomplete, try to hear if it begins a musical thought or ends a musical thought (more on "musical thoughts" in a moment). Also, if you listen really hard, you should hear that the **count 1** usually has a tiny bit more of an accent than the **count 5**.

TIP: In some music, the **count 1** of a new major phrase of music will have a very strong accent (or, at least, an accent that's stronger than the other **count 1s**). While this won't happen in all music, it happens enough that it's worth paying attention to. Also, it helps to listen for the transition between two major phrases. If you can hear the resolution or conclusion of a major phrase—likely to be a handful of beats, not just one beat—that will prep you to listen for the beginning of the next major phrase, which will be a **count 1**. Take the example of a verse ending and the chorus beginning, which is a transition between two major phrases. The first beat of the chorus will be a **count 1**.

2) *Listen for a mini-phrase (set of 8) of music.* While an accent is a specific beat of music, a set of 8 is composed of multiple beats. So a set of 8 as a whole may seem less precise or more vague to your ears than an accent. You have to try to develop a sense for them because sets of 8 hit you more at an intuitive level.

It's hard to put into words what a set of 8 sounds like. Typically, a set of 8, like a sentence of words, will stand out in some way. It'll have integrity, like a sentence of words has integrity. You'll hear a theme or what I describe as a "musical thought." (Remember, these smaller themes then come together to form bigger themes, which are the major phrases.)

So, in the same way that a written sentence pops out a little—through structure, theme and integrity—a set of 8 does, too. Over eight beats of music you might hear things such as a:

- Setup and resolution.

- "Call and response," which is when the music makes a statement and then there's an answer or reaction to the statement.

- Beginning point and an ending point; or maybe just a beginning point.

Also, listen for some sort of transition between sets of 8, like something coming to an end, which would tip you off that something new is about to begin.

As you listen for all these elements, try to listen to the music as a whole and get a feel for the bigger structure. When you feel something about to begin...get ready...start counting!

While themes can be subtle and tricky, they can also be easy to hear. The two songs earlier in this chapter are good examples of songs with an easy-to-hear structure and theme ("Brother Louie," video 1.1; and "Gotta Do Some War Work, Baby," video 1.2; plus, I count the sets of 8 for both songs in video 1.5). Each set of 8 stands out as a musical thought with integrity. Go back and listen to the themes of the sets of 8 in those songs to see if they reveal a **count 1** and when to begin counting. While most songs are not this easy, there are plenty of songs that are almost as obvious.

TIP: The first four-beat measure in a set of 8 is called the *heavy measure;* and the second four-beat measure is called the *light measure* (terms courtesy of dance educator Skippy Blair). In some music, the first measure actually has a "heaviness" to it when compared to the second measure, which will sound "lighter." You may hear this in *some* music, not in *all* music.

TIP: I suggest you don't get hung-up on a hard song, especially as a beginner. Curveballs are common. I'm never surprised when I hear something confusing. When I get lost, and I still do, I simply declare it difficult music and move on. I often capture the name of the song for later, then I let it go. I'll talk more about hard music in Chapter 2.

Even though I've given you specific things to listen for—accents and mini-phrases (sets of 8)—don't try to label what you hear. Music can move by quickly and you may not always know what you just heard, but you heard something and it may help to reveal the sets of 8. The "clues" will vary from song to song, so there really isn't one way to hear the sets of 8. In fact, as soon as you think you've found a rule for hearing the sets of 8, you'll find exceptions to that rule. Instead, just listen *actively* and take it all in.

From now on, whenever and wherever you hear music, count the sets of 8. Make it a habit. The more you work at it, the more natural it'll become. Even if you don't think you're making progress, you're slowly training your ear. Have faith that your brain knows what's going on.

COUNTING ALERT: When I was learning to dance I was bombarded by different ways to count, which led to confusion and paralysis. Let me explain. Part of my confusion came from not knowing the difference between the musician's count (counted in **4s**) and the dancer's count (counted in **8s**). Another part of my confusion came from not understanding that, although related, there's a difference between *counting music* and *counting a step pattern* (a **step pattern** is a dance figure or dance step). And another part of my confusion was because dance teachers counted in different ways and in confusing ways (there are bad ways for dancers to count a step pattern; for example, counting weight changes). So, be aware that you may hear different ways to count. In general, if you butt heads with some weird counting, just roll with it. Ask for clarification and try to convert it into what you know. SHAMELESS PLUG ALERT: This is a book about counting music, not dance. If you're learning to dance, it's good to know how to count a step pattern (the **pattern count**). Check out Chapter 6, "Counting Step Patterns," in my book *Every Man's Survival Guide to Ballroom Dancing* (iHateToDance.com). Counting music is something you practice off the dance floor, like when you watch others dance or when you listen casually. If you're dancing, you're probably counting a step pattern in your head.

Music creates order out of chaos.

— YEHUDI MENUHIN,
VIOLINIST AND CONDUCTOR

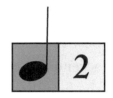

Practice Counting Music

THE MUSIC IS WHIZZING BY YOU. Maybe it's bold, with accents all over the place. Or maybe it's subtle, with nothing to grab onto. Maybe it's wild. Maybe it's eclectic. Or maybe it just sounds totally random. Where to begin?

Even if you hear no order to music, there's order. And it's probably a high degree of order. The best way to identify and connect to this order is to count. Once you see how it's done, you might be surprised how quickly you pick it up. So let's hop over to the web page, stream a few tunes and count. Then we'll look at a piece of harder music, a song by Adele. I'll finish this chapter with tips on practicing.

Go to HearTheBeatFeelTheMusic.com and watch the **video series 2.1**, "Count Music–Sets of 8." It's a bunch of videos of me counting sets of 8 to a variety of music. Have at it. I've included some salsa music, too. Salsa can be difficult because there's a lot of percussion, which can be confusing. Plus, salsa is uptempo, which means everything hits you faster so there's less time to process what you hear.

POP QUIZ: Here's a song whose chorus has a very accented beat. This accented beat keeps repeating. On that beat the vocal is strongly accented with the word "hey." This accented "hey" is in each set of 8 of the chorus (actually, just the first three sets of 8, not the fourth). The song starts with the chorus so you'll hear three "heys" in the first 10 seconds. The song is "Little Talks" by Of Monsters and Men. Your challenge is to identify which count is getting the accented "hey" (**count 1** or **count 2** or **count 3**, etc.). Go to the website and watch **video 2.2**. For the answer, go to the last page of the book, which is the last page of Chapter 7. I also count the phrasing for this song in **video 6.2.1**.

HAND EXERCISE: Here's a simple hand exercise you can do when you count sets of 8 to help bring the count into your body. It's also a good way to visually identify the sets of 8 for a group of people, so I use it when I teach. All you do is chop or punch out each beat of music with your hand. First, chop out **counts 1** to **4** with one hand; then chop out **counts 5** to **8** with the other hand. This gets your body moving on each beat. Plus, it helps with timing and coordination because your hand can't be late. Also, switching hands between measures on **count 5** gets you to acknowledge the four-beat measures in the music. Have a look at how it's done by the master, Skippy Blair. I'm honored to have Skippy, the teacher who taught me how to connect to music, demonstrate this. Go to the website and watch **video 2.3**, "Count Music–Hand Exercise by Skippy Blair."

CLUB DANCING TIP: Even you hip-hoppers, club-dancers and freestylers will benefit from understanding **count 1**. Start new moves on **count 1** or **count 5**; then start the next new move on the next **count 1**. It'll improve your connection to the music and make you a better dancer, and you'll enjoy it more.

TIP: There are people with musical talent who don't have to count. They never had to count. They naturally feel the music. They may question why you're counting and make offhand remarks about it. Ignore them! You can learn to hear the beat through counting. If you stick with it, eventually you'll feel it too.

Easy Versus Hard Music

I often say that there's easy music and there's hard music. Both are common. The music in this chapter has been mostly on the easy side. If you do partner dancing or club dancing or dance fitness (Zumba, aerobics, etc.), the music will usually be easy. The background music at your gym, and workout music in general, should be on the easy side.

The problem, dang it, is that there are songs out there with all kinds of weird stuff going on. Trying to hear the sets of 8 in difficult music may very well twist your brain into a knot. For that reason, especially in the beginning, you need to stick to easy music, music where the sets of 8 pop out a little. I talk more about handling hard music in the third bullet point on practicing at the end of this chapter.

When you encounter difficult music and get lost, try to listen to the percussion. That's because—I said this before but it needs repeating—*the percussion section of the band establishes the underlying beat of music.* You'll be tempted or distracted a lot by the melody and vocals, but melody and vocals can be misleading. You need to listen to the drums!

Identifying the percussion or rhythm section (drums, percussion, keyboard and string instruments) is not easy. Note that some instruments, like guitar and piano, can play both melody and rhythm, so it can be tricky. And even if you can identify the rhythm section, it still may not reveal the sets of 8, but at least you've proceeded in a logical way.

There are a number of reasons why a song might be difficult. Let's listen to one example, "Rolling in the Deep" by Adele. I find this song instructive because it has some sets of 8 that are easy to hear and some that are hard to hear. To my ear, the easy sets of 8 are clear and stand out without the need to count. But the hard sets of 8 are so tricky that unless I concentrate I get lost. The hard sets of 8 are difficult because the vocals do not line up with the sets of 8. Adele's "vocal phrasing" becomes complex and this complexity contributes a lot to making it a great song.

Go to the website and watch **video 2.4**, "Hear Sets of 8–Easy Versus Hard Music." We're just going to listen to the beginning of the song, the first one minute and 20 seconds, which will be four major phrases of music. Each major phrase will have four sets of 8.

In the video, I'll identify the major phrases by using a "musical skeleton," which you'll learn more about in Chapter 6. But it's quite simple, really. A set of 8 is noted by the numeral "8" like this: 8. And a major phrase that's made up of four sets of 8 is noted like this: 8888. So the musical skeleton for the first four major phrases look like this:

8888
8888
8888 – *hard!*
8888

It's the third major phrase that's hard. It runs from 0:44 to 1:02 and is denoted in the musical skeleton above with the word "*hard.*" Even if you're dialed into the sets of 8 in the first major phrase (0:07–0:25) and second major phrase (0:26–0:43), starting at 0:44 you may lose it unless you concentrate. The fourth major phrase is the chorus, which runs from 1:03 to 1:20, and it has sets of 8 that are easy to hear. The first six seconds of the song are a quick intro, which you can ignore.

The first time through, close your eyes and see if you can count or naturally hear the sets of 8 and major phrases without counting. Whether you count or not, I want you to feel what happens when the song becomes complex in the third major phrase at the 0:44 mark. TIP: The key to counting the third major phrase is to listen more to the percussion and less to Adele's vocals.

Practice

Practice is the hardest part of learning, and training is the essence of transformation.
— Ann Voskamp, writer

Getting to know music at the intuitive level takes time. Don't expect a switch to flip in your brain from "no rhythm" to "rhythm." It'll be more like a dial where the more you train, the better you get. And it'll only happen through training. Since you probably listen to music all the time, the real effort is remembering to practice.

- Practicing shouldn't be a big deal. As you listen to a song, challenge yourself: *Gee, I wonder if I can count the sets of 8 and identify the beat?* Then listen for 10 or 20 seconds, and when you think you hear a **count 1**, start counting the sets of 8. Count for another 20 or 30 seconds, and either you're counting correctly or you're not. If you blow it the first time, try again. Then move on, either counting the next song or going back to vegging-out to the music. That's it and it only took a minute. I hope you find this fun, especially as you start getting better at it.

- Practice anytime and anywhere you hear music. I love challenging myself with new music. I always listen to background music, whether I'm at a café, a store, an event, a friend's place, or on an elevator—you name it. Practice on your commute to work, or at the gym, or as you drift off to sleep at night. When I was deeply into it, I'd try to count the background music in movies or on TV (that's often difficult music).

- As you know, I crudely group music into two categories: music with a beat that's *easy* to hear and music with a beat that's *hard* to hear. And I'll keep saying: *you have to hear the sets of 8 in easy music before you can hear them in the harder stuff.* If you're stumped after 30 or 40 seconds of listening to a song, assume that it's hard music and move on to another song. Don't get bogged down trying to figure out one piece of difficult music. But if you can, capture the title of the song and save it for later when you can play it to a teacher or friend who can help you hear the sets of 8. There are smartphone apps, like SoundHound and Shazam, which are amazing at identifying the names of songs.

- You need to go out of your way to try new music, because getting variety will improve your ability to handle all kinds of music. Don't just listen to music in your music collection. Vast amounts of music can be searched for free on the web (search for "best music websites"). I like YouTube, Pandora and Spotify for browsing (Spotify has a monthly fee). Remember radios? You can get a lot of variety by surfing the radio dial. When I was training myself back in the 1990s I used to bounce rapidly around the dial as an informal way to test myself on a variety of music, particularly musical genres that I didn't normally listen to.

- There will always be difficult songs within a genre but you should be able to find easy music in most of the popular genres. Initially, I'd try stuff like rock, pop, hip-hop, rap and R & B. Electronic dance music—like house, techno, dance, etc.—should be good because dancers like easy music. Blues is good. Jazz should be good, but there's some jazz, like a subgenre called bebop (think Dizzy Gillespie and Miles Davis), which will have some challenging songs. I'd stay away from salsa music in the very beginning because of the fast tempo and overwhelming percussion. Latin music with a slower tempo should be okay (more on tempo in Chapter 5). Classical music would not be a good place to start. Take a pass on Gregorian chanting and Native American flute music or anything that doesn't have a drum section. In general, if you can't hear the drums, you're probably dealing with harder music.

- If you're struggling to hear the sets of 8, get confirmation from others to make sure you're counting correctly. I know, this is a wild card because I'm asking you to involve other people. Find someone who can hear the sets of 8, not just four-beat measures. "Testing" can take as little as a minute of listening together to one song, so you're not asking much. I used to ask my dance teachers after classes and it would only take about 30 seconds to count a few sets of 8 to the background music. I also used to ask strangers at dances and they were happy to help. If you have the chance, play the difficult songs you've collected to someone and have them count the sets of 8. One way or another, try to get feedback, because if you're counting incorrectly, you'll just reinforce the error. As dance educator Skippy Blair likes to say: "Practice makes permanent. Only perfect practice makes perfect."

Your goal should be 100 percent confidence in hearing the **8s**, even if your accuracy is less than 100 percent (music can be tricky, so you may not always be right). It's easy to guess at a piece of music and be correct. So get a feel for your confidence level. Ask yourself: *To what degree am I guessing?* When you're confident, there's no guessing, you just know.

If you don't have any prior training or natural ability in music, hearing the sets of 8 will take time. Plan on weeks or months before you're confident with all types of music. Although it took me about two years of training, I was actually pretty good at it after six months. A lot of the additional months were spent working on difficult music and bringing the beat into my body so I didn't have to think about it.

Practice, experiment, persist, and you'll improve.

NOTES

*For those of you in the cheap seats
I'd like ya to clap your hands to this one;
the rest of you can just rattle your jewelry!*

— JOHN LENNON

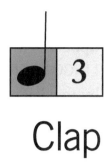

Clap

YOU'RE AT A CONCERT and the crowd begins to clap. But the guy on your left claps differently than the gal on your right. You look around and there's no consensus. Everyone is clapping differently! What's up with that?

While clapping to music is simple, in practice it's a bit messy. Fear not, we will make mincemeat of this messiness. And you will reap the benefits because learning to clap will:

- Help you to hear the sets of 8 and feel the beat.

- Improve your overall connection to music.

- Get your body moving to music.

- Help you save face, because in an audience people may judge your clapping. Clapping can be a test of your rhythm, so you may as well do it right—or people will know you ain't got no rhythm.

Before we clap, a couple of definitions: The **downbeat** is the odd-numbered beat, on **counts 1, 3, 5** and **7**. The **upbeat** is the even-numbered beat, on **counts 2, 4, 6** and **8**. LINGO ALERT: *Downbeat* and *upbeat* are defined differently by musicians. And you'll hear other terms used to label *downbeat* and *upbeat*. It's confusing. When you hear these words, note the source and take them in context.

On Which Beats Do You Clap?

Let's look at the three most common choices for clapping. Which do you think is correct?

1. You could clap on every beat, **counts 1, 2, 3, 4, 5, 6, 7** and **8**.

2. You could clap on the downbeat (**counts 1, 3, 5** and **7**).

3. You could clap on the upbeat (**counts 2, 4, 6** and **8**).

In America, people in the know—musicians, dancers, hepcats—clap on the upbeat, **counts 2, 4, 6** and **8**. If you're feeling the music, it's going to feel best to clap on the upbeat. Granted, this may be conditioning based on American culture, but that's the way it is.

Not so fast…I need a little wiggle room. First, not all music makes you want to clap. For example, salsa music will probably not make you want to clap. Second, there may be songs that are exceptions (hard to come up with any, but one would be Elton John's "Benny and the Jets," where the clapping is on every beat—note that it's from Great Britain).

Third, if your background in music has *not* been typically American, you may feel the music and where to clap differently. Fourth, you may be in an audience and a member of the band starts you clapping on something other than **2, 4, 6** and **8** (most likely, on every beat).

Still, the safest rule of thumb is to clap on **2, 4, 6** and **8**. Although this may not be universal, it's ingrained enough in America that you can even buy T-shirts on the web that read: "Friends don't let friends clap on **1** and **3**."

Follow the Crowd?

It's a funny thing but audiences often clap incorrectly. They sometimes clap on every beat and they sometimes clap on **counts 1, 3, 5** and **7**. Often an audience is mixed and not everybody is clapping in sync. This is not hard to see on TV or in YouTube videos when the camera shoots the audience during a music performance.

Also, sometimes people clap off-time (i.e., not precisely on the beat). Or, as they clap, they speed up or slow down (i.e., change the tempo). If it's a live performance, that can throw off the band's performance. I've read discussions online by band members on how audiences can screw up a band's timing. But bands also like it when the audience claps, even if it's not perfect clapping, because it lets the band know that you're into the song. Clapping builds energy, participation and community, which adds to the performance. Clapping is not an audience participation gimmick. Your hands are a percussion instrument and you become part of the performance.

So, if you're in an audience, glance around and have some awareness of what the audience is doing. Are they all clapping together? Don't be afraid to clap against the group if you know you're right. If you're new to clapping, question your accuracy. Remember, you have witnesses.

The Secret to Clapping

If there's a secret to clapping, it's recognizing another common pattern in popular music: the natural pairing of beats. This two-beat pattern consists of one *downbeat* and one *upbeat*, and it keeps repeating. So **counts 1** and **2** are the first pair, **counts 3** and **4** are the second pair, and so on.

This pairing will be obvious in some music, less obvious in some music and absent in some music. Sometimes you'll barely hear it, and sometimes you can't hear it at all but you know it's there. Like sets of 8, the pairing of beats is just "in" the music.

While you won't hear the pairing of beats in all music, I think it occurs enough in popular music that it's a pattern you should know. If you can hear the natural pairing of beats, it will tell you instantly where to clap—on the second beat of the pair, the upbeat—without the need to count the sets of 8.

Here's what to listen for (this is not a rule, it's just a place to start): If the pairing is easy to hear then it often, but not always, sounds like a deeper-pitched downbeat (**counts 1, 3, 5** and **7**) followed by a higher-pitched upbeat (**counts 2, 4, 6** and **8**). Sometimes the upbeats almost have a lifting feeling. To my ear, two beats often sound like "boom tick." These sounds, "boom" and "tick," are just my words for a deeper-pitched sound and a higher-pitched sound, respectively (you can use whatever words you like, even nonsense syllables, which is known as *scat* in jazz singing). If the "tick" has an emphasis, I note it in all caps, so two beats would be "boom TICK."

It's easy to hear the pairing of beats in many popular genres of music like blues, rock, rap, pop and electronic dance music (EDM). To get you warmed up, here's a video I made a few years back in which I identify downbeats and upbeats in some popular music. Go to HearTheBeatFeelTheMusic.com and watch **video 3.1**, "Hear the Downbeat and Upbeat in Dance Music."

NOTATION ALERT: When I notate eight beats of music, I break them into two-beat increments by using double hyphens. For example, eight beats of music with an emphasis on **counts 2, 4, 6** and **8** looks like this:

boom TICK—boom TICK—boom TICK—boom TICK

THE "STOMP-CLAP" EXERCISE: This exercise will give you a feel for the pairing of beats. I have a memory from childhood of watching old-timey washboard bands. Sometimes one band member would act as the drum section by first stomping his foot and then clapping his hands. The stomp was the downbeat and the clap was the upbeat. So eight beats of music would look like this:

stomp CLAP—stomp CLAP—stomp CLAP—stomp CLAP

Do the following three variations and compare them. Do them with no music and all at the same tempo, which is kind of slow:

1. Do a stomp and a CLAP and keep repeating it. Get into it. Stop.

2. Just stomp your foot and get into it. Groove a little. Stop.

3. Just clap and get into that. Keep grooving. Stop.

How did they feel? In which of the three variations did you feel the most rhythmic, like you were an instrument? It's subtle, so keep your expectations low. Try it again and don't think too hard. Try it also to some music and see how that feels. For me, both "stomp stomp" and "CLAP CLAP" make me feel like a metronome. But "stomp CLAP" makes me feel like I'm a set of drums.

HOW TO FAKE MUSICAL TALENT: If you ever hang out with friends who sing or play guitar, doing a "stomp CLAP" in the background will create a drum track for the musicians. It's fun and a good way to fake musical talent. Seriously, it works.

COOL TRICK: Here's another thing that may help you get a feel for the pairing of beats. It's a YouTube video on how to "beatbox," the art of producing drum sounds with your voice. If you've never been exposed to beatboxing you may find this odd. Try not to think of it as singing. Think of the instructor's voice as a set of drums, which is creating a drum track. To create a downbeat and an upbeat, the instructor uses the phrase "bouncing CATS." If you repeat that phrase over and over in sort of a breathy voice, you create a drum track with your voice. The "b" in bouncing becomes the downbeat, and the "C" in CATS becomes the upbeat. Watch him do it in the video. It's about a five-minute video that goes through a variety of stuff, but the demo of "bouncing CATS" runs for just a few seconds from 0:53 to 1:06. Go to the website and watch **video 3.2**, "Beat Boxing Basics with Dub FX." Of course, listen to the whole video and explore your inner beatboxer.

DANCING TIP: The thing I love about the downbeat and upbeat is that it helps me to *feel* the beat, to bring it from my head and into my body. When it's in the music, the pairing of beats is a distinctive pulse, which is easy to grab onto. When moving to music, it acts like an autopilot and keeps me on the beat. My goal is to be *entrained* by the music—to be mesmerized, spellbound—and connecting to the simple, repetitive pattern of the downbeat and upbeat helps (more on *entrainment* in Chapter 7).

TIP: Here's another thing I love about the pairing of beats: Two beats hit my ear faster than eight beats. Sometimes the pairing of beats is all I need to identify the beat. If I'm not 100 percent sure, within another eight beats I'll hear a **count 1,** then I'll hear a set of 8 and it all gets confirmed. So hearing the downbeat and upbeat can be one of the first clues and one of the best clues to help me hear the beat.

More Clapping Exercises

START CLAPPING: Clapping is another thing to practice as you listen to music throughout the day. One way to practice is this: When a song starts, don't count. Instead, jump in and clap whenever it feels right. Once you get into the song and think you're right, then count the sets of 8 and check your work. Are you clapping on the **2, 4, 6** and **8**? By the way, you don't really have to clap. You can softly snap your fingers or gently slap your thigh. You can even do this standing in line at the post office.

LISTEN TO FINGER-SNAPPING: Snapping your fingers to music is similar to clapping. There are a handful of songs with snapping on the upbeat as part of the percussion section. One of the classics is the 1964 number-one hit "King of the Road" by Roger Miller. While the snapping continues throughout the song, in the first 16 beats it's about the only thing you hear. It's a great hook.

But if you listen closely, you can also hear a deep, soft base string on **counts 1, 3, 5** and **7**. The snapping is on **2, 4, 6** and **8**. I describe the pattern for a set of 8 like this:

boom SNAP—boom SNAP—boom SNAP—boom SNAP

Go to the website and watch **video 3.3**, "King of the Road." Count the sets of 8 to the first 16 beats a few times. Try to really get into the finger-snapping in those first 16 beats. *Feel how a simple snap can create rhythm and structure.* I also count the snapping for you in the next video, **video 3.4**. It's the first song.

LISTEN TO MORE FINGER-SNAPPING: The first time through this video, close your eyes so you can't see my finger count the sets of 8. As you listen, relax and let the music wash over you, because that will help your right brain—your intuitive and creative mind—to connect. Ponder this notion of the natural pairing of beats: a deeper-pitched downbeat (the "boom") followed by a higher-pitched upbeat (the "SNAP"). Still with your eyes closed, try to feel the sets of 8 without counting. Go to the playlist and watch **video 3.4**, "Where to Snap Your Fingers in Music," for a compilation of songs with snapping.

LISTEN TO CLAPPING: There are many songs with clapping (real clapping or electronically synthesized) as part of the song. The first time through the following cuts, close your eyes (so you can't see me counting) and count the sets of 8 to confirm that the clapping is on the upbeat. Go to the playlist and watch **video 3.5**, "Where to Clap in Music."

WATCH PEOPLE CLAPPING: Here's a video of people clapping correctly. I thought it would be good to see it in action to add some depth. In America, the early roots of clapping on the upbeat came from jazz and gospel music. A group that keeps early jazz music (big band era, 1930s to 1940s) alive is the Lindy Hop swing dance community. They know their music and they like to clap, especially in a "jam circle" (the group forms a circle and couples take their turn in the middle to show off their stuff).

Check out the audience clapping in this fun video of a jam circle. Count the sets of 8 and confirm that they're clapping on the upbeat. This is harder music to count because the tempo is fast, the beat is soft and it's not a perfect recording, but the thematic structure of the sets of 8 is strong. Go to the playlist and watch **video 3.6**, "Clap to Music–Lindy Hop Jam Circle."

GET YOUR SNAP AND CLAP ON: This video is Feist performing "One Evening." I've included this video to give you an example of an artist who engages her audience to both snap and clap; plus, it's a good song for practicing your snapping and clapping. She starts the song by snapping her fingers on the upbeat to get the audience snapping, which they do. Then the snapping fades. Then, at 3:27 minutes, she starts clapping on the upbeat and the audience joins her by clapping. Then the clapping fades.

Go to the playlist and watch **video 3.7**, "One Evening" by Feist. Your mission is to snap or clap through the entire song and stay on the upbeat, which you can check at the 3:27 minute mark. This is a good practice song because it's challenging. Even though I think the sets of 8 and phrasing are a little tricky, I'm confident about the beat because I hear the rhythmic pairing of beats through most of the song.

POP QUIZ: Let's finish this chapter with another example of an audience clapping to music, which you can use to sharpen and test your ear. The hitch is that, initially, the audience claps incorrectly on the downbeat. What's fascinating is that the artist, Harry Connick, Jr., does something about it. At some point he deletes a beat of music, which makes the audience, unwittingly, shift their clapping to the upbeat. Your job is to identify the point in the music (note the time in the progress bar) when that shift occurs. You can find the answer (and some entertaining discussion) if you read the comments on the YouTube page below the video. Or the answer is at the end of Chapter 7. Go to the playlist and watch **video 3.8**, "Harry Connick, Jr., and Clapping." (TRIVIA ALERT: And then there was the time that Neil Young playfully called out his audience for clapping off-time. Just google "Neil Young" and "clapping" if you want to watch a bad quality cell phone recording of the incident.)

The benefits of clapping can be subtle so don't expect miracles. But learning to clap on the upbeat will help you feel the beat and connect to the music.

The effect of music is so very much more powerful and penetrating than is that of the other arts, for these others speak only of the shadow, but music of the essence.

— ARTHUR SCHOPENHAUER

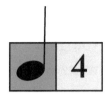

Waltz

A WALTZ...WHAT'S NOT TO LIKE? But the waltz is a different kind of animal. It's unlike all the music you've listened to so far.

So what's the big deal? The waltz is counted in *sets of 6* versus *sets of 8*. That's all you need to know for now to understand a waltz, because beyond that it gets a little geeky. But I'd be letting you down by offering no explanation. So, in the second half of this chapter, I discuss a bit of the music theory behind the waltz, specifically *time signatures*, because that's a phrase that gets thrown around a lot.

When I was first learning how to hear the beat with no one to guide me, this is how I identified a waltz: I always assumed a piece of music was in sets of 8 (not a waltz). I would try to count sets of 8 for 20 or 30 seconds. If that didn't work, yet I was sure I could hear the beat, I tried counting sets of 6. That usually worked. If I couldn't count sets of 6 or sets of 8, I'd move on quickly to easier music. I still think this is an acceptable strategy for a beginner.

But let's add something. Let's amp up your awareness of a waltz. Let's get into the groove of a waltz so that once you gain a knack for it, you should be able to recognize a waltz without counting. This won't be hard because a waltz has a different feel to it than music structured in sets of 8.

What does a waltz feel like? A waltz has a "down up up" feeling over three beats of music, which keeps repeating. A simple way I sometimes describe this feeling is "oom-pah-pah" (from the "Oom-Pah-Pah" song in the musical *Oliver*).

Wait, stop…you said a waltz is in sets of 6! Correct, so over six beats of music the feeling will be "down up up, down up up." Like sets of 8, sets of 6 will often sound like a "sentence" of music. Sets of 6 can be heard because they're "in" the music. A set of 6 is also known as a six-beat *miniphrase* of music.

When counting a waltz, non-musicians (that's you and me) should do it like this: **1 2 3—4 5 6**. I know, musicians will disagree because they count a waltz like this: **1 2 3— 1 2 3**. Both ways are correct, it just depends upon who you are and what you're doing. Musicians create a waltz in three-beat measures, so that's the way they think. But dancers think in mini-phrases (sets of 6), which recognize that measures usually come in pairs, because that's the structure they use to choreograph a dance. You can translate the musician's count into the dancer's count by recognizing that **count 1** of the second measure is the same as **count 4** in a set of 6. It looks like this:

1 2 3   4 5 6 – dancer's count (*set of 6*)
1 2 3   1 2 3 – musician's count (two three-beat *measures*)

A few more things to note about a waltz: First, often, but not always, **count 1** and **count 4**, the first beat of each measure in a set of 6, have an accent or emphasis. Second, note that a three-beat measure is structured *downbeat upbeat upbeat*, which aligns with the "down up up" feeling. Also note that waltz music will not make you want to clap.

DANCING TIP: When you dance a waltz with a "down up up" feeling, your head and body go down slightly on the downbeats (**count 1, count 4**) and up on the upbeats (**counts 2** and **3, counts 5** and **6**). This is referred to as the "rise and fall," and it helps define the look, feel and style of the dance.

How common is a waltz? For me, in a day of listening to music, I might not hear a waltz at all. Or I might hear it one or two or three times. Whether you hear it every day or not, it happens enough that you need to know it. Plus, it's an important category of music and, arguably, there's a cultural significance to the waltz.

Waltzes cross many genres of music. You can find waltzes in classical, jazz, rock 'n' roll, country, Latin, tango and more. Many well-known songs are waltzes. The national anthem of the United States, "The Star-Spangled Banner," is a waltz. If you're a fan of the movie *The Godfather*, you'll recognize the theme song, "Godfather Waltz." The tempo for waltzes can range from very slow to very fast. It's not uncommon for a wedding couple to choose a waltz for their first dance because there are many slow, romantic waltzes. Fast waltzes are often for dancing a Viennese waltz. The waltz is the oldest ballroom dance, dating back to the 1700s.

Let's dig into some waltz music. Maybe, just maybe, your "inner Johann Strauss" (TRIVIA ALERT: composer of over 400 waltzes, including the "The Blue Danube") will latch on to the structure and the feel of a waltz. Since a good number of popular songs are waltzes, ask yourself this question: *Am I already familiar with the waltz but didn't know it?*

Go to HearTheBeatFeelTheMusic.com and watch **video 4.1**, "A Medley of Waltz Music." It's just clips of different waltzes, with no counting. Try to pick up on the vibe of a waltz. Then, watch me count sets of 6 in **video 4.2**, "Count Waltz Music–Sets of 6." TIP: As you listen to waltzes to train your ear, let your head and shoulders drop a little on **counts 1** and **4** to help you get into the down-up-up feeling. Try to bring the waltz into your body.

The Waltz and Time Signatures

Sets of 8, sets of 6…sets of X? Is there more?

Yes, sometimes music is structured in other groupings. Enter the world of *time signatures*.

I've avoided talking about time signatures because they're a part of music theory, which can be complicated and TMI (too much information). Understanding time signatures is not necessary to hear the beat and enjoy music. I'm officially labeling the rest of this chapter with an ADVANCED INFO ALERT. So, proceed with that understanding, and if it's confusing, just skim through it.

Here's a short discussion of the time signature. All I'm going to do is describe it and show you how it converts into what you've learned already.

Time signature is a system of musical notation that identifies the *meter* of the music. There, I said it, no big deal.

On a piece of sheet music the time signature is denoted by the two stacked numbers to the far left, which look like a fraction, like 2/4, 3/4, 4/4, 5/4, 6/8, 12/8, etc. The top number is what interests us the most because it tells us how many beats there are to a *measure*, which translates directly to how you count the music. For our purposes, there are only two time signatures of importance:

- **The 4/4 time signature**, which is four beats to a measure so the top number is "4." The overwhelming majority of popular, mainstream Western music is in the 4/4 time signature. All the music we've been listening to in prior chapters, which is music that gets counted in sets of 8 because measures are paired, is in the 4/4 time signature (except one song, explained in the MUSIC NOTE below).

- **The 3/4 time signature,** which is three beats to a measure so the top number is "3." A waltz is in 3/4 time. This is probably the next most popular time signature, but it's still used for only a tiny amount of music compared to 4/4 time.

LINGO ALERT: When referring to a time signature the word "signature" is often dropped. So a common way to verbally describe them would be "three-four time" for the 3/4 time signature and "four-four time" for the 4/4 time signature.

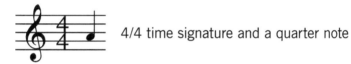

4/4 time signature and a quarter note

The bottom number of the fraction of the time signature—the number "4" in the case of both 3/4 time and 4/4 time—tells you what kind of note…whoops, I know, things just got fuzzy. But don't stress, keep reading.

I find the bottom number important for one particular reason. It's the explanation behind a term you might occasionally hear: *quarter note.* When the bottom number is a "4" that means it's a quarter note. Although quarter note is a part of music theory, you might hear it used in a dance class because it's not uncommon for a dance teacher to also be a musician. So it wouldn't hurt to tack the phrase quarter note on the back wall of your brain for occasional access.

SUPER-ADVANCED INFO ALERT: I probably shouldn't define it any further because you don't need to know this, but here goes: a *quarter note* is a musical note with the time value of one quarter of a whole note. Now take a deep breath and just let it go.

Here's the thing to know about a quarter note: *what a non-musician would call the "beat," a musician might call a "quarter note."* So, whenever you hear someone talk about a quarter note, don't freak out, just consider that they may be talking about the beat of music. For example, if someone says, "clap on the quarter note," they may just mean, "clap on the beat." If someone throws "eighth note" or "sixteenth note" at you... duck. But, seriously, that's way, way TMI if your only goal is to hear the beat. I think musicians mean well when they throw terms like quarter note and eighth note at the masses of starving non-musicians, but really, it's confusing.

My apologies to music mavens if I took liberties and oversimplified time signatures. But, hey, that's my job, to uncomplicate the complicated and comfort the confused.

LINGO ALERT: Generally, "3/4 time" and "waltz time" are used synonymously (although not all 3/4 time music will make you feel like dancing a waltz).

ULTRA-ADVANCED INFO ALERT: This may be TMI, but I think a chapter on the waltz and time signatures might be lacking if I didn't mention the 6/8 time signature because you occasionally find it in popular music. The oddball thing about this time signature is that there's both a fast way to count it, in sets of 6 like a waltz, plus a slow way to count it, as if it were in sets of 8. Pretty trippy, huh? Even though 6/8 time is, technically, not waltz timing, it can feel like a waltz and people often dance a Viennese waltz (a fast waltz). There are a few well-known songs in 6/8 time; for example, "One and Only" by Adele, "Kiss from a Rose" by Seal, "Iris" by Goo Goo Dolls, "We Are the Champions" by Queen and "Norwegian Wood" by the Beatles.

MUSIC NOTE: I revealed in Chapter 1 that there was something different about the song "Dark Love" (video 1.4 and video 1.5, the third song). It's actually in the 12/8 time signature and, I confess, I initially missed it. To keep things simple, I wanted to use only 4/4 time and 3/4 time music in this book. But I decided to include this song anyway because it's an example of trickier music and it illustrates a point: sometimes you get an uncommon time signature that can still be counted in sets of 8. In my experience, often the 2/4 time signature can also be counted in sets of 8 (but that's not a rule, it's just my experience).

There are many uncommon time signatures, but they're rare in popular music so I say, no worries. For example, Dave Brubeck's jazz piece "Take Five," which is in 5/4 time, is often cited as a piece of popular music that's in an uncommon time signature. It was a top hit way back in 1961 and it's still popular today.

Still, you may run into weird stuff. When I hit a song and I get stumped—that is, I can't count sets of 6 or sets of 8—I go through the following routine because I want to know if my counting was faulty or if it's an uncommon time signature. I google the name of the song, plus the phrase "time signature" or "sheet music." Sometimes I find the time signature mentioned in a discussion. Or I can usually find the first page of the sheet music. Then I look at the time signature, which is the fraction on the left. If it's an odd time signature, I might try to count it, just to test myself. If it's 3/4 or 4/4 time, I'll go back and try harder to count the **6s** or **8s**, respectively.

There will always be an occasional piece of unusual music that will confound and befuddle the best. Sometimes it's an unusual time signature. Sometimes a song uses multiple time signatures (e.g., "Money" by Pink Floyd and "Lucy in the Sky with Diamonds" by the Beatles). Sometimes the rhythm section is not there, or it's so soft or complex that you can't hear any grouping of beats. When this happens, you'll get lost. But don't fret; it's not your fault. Just smile and move on.

Virtually every writer I know would rather be a musician.

— KURT VONNEGUT

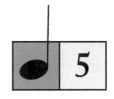

Tempo

Some psychologists have suggested that people have an innate preference for rhythms at a frequency of two hertz, which is equivalent to 120 beats per minute (bpm), or two beats per second. When asked to tap their fingers or walk, many people unconsciously settle into a rhythm of 120 bpm. And an analysis of more than 74,000 popular songs produced between 1960 and 1990 found that 120 bpm was the most prevalent pulse.

— Ferris Jabr, "Let's Get Physical: The Psychology of Effective Workout Music" http://www.scientific american.com/article/psychology-workout-music

WELCOME TO THE EASIEST chapter in the book, I think.

Let's get the definition out of the way. **Tempo** is the speed of the music. It's the speed of the *underlying beat*. It's measured in beats per minute, or bpm for short, like 120 bpm.

While tempo is not directly related to hearing the beat, it might come into play. For example, with a fast tempo it may be harder to hear the beat because the information hits you faster. But an extremely slow tempo could be hard, too, because, well, it's so darn slow, which is not what you're expecting (it's especially hard if the drum section is soft and the melody or lyrics is distracting).

Still, getting a sense of the tempo will improve your connection to music because tempo contributes a lot to the feel and energy. If you dance or work out to music, I think having an awareness of tempo will give you an edge. For example, as you get to know tempo you may find that you like a specific tempo for dancing or working out. So be on the lookout for "your tempo" (a concept courtesy of Skippy Blair).

I don't know what it is about tempo, but I feel more confident around music when I have a sense of the tempo, or know the tempo, or know that I can calculate it in a matter of seconds. I've calculated the tempo for most of the songs on my computer. This lets me organize my music by tempo, which helps when creating playlists for dancing and working out, and when I want to create a mood, like for a dinner party.

Tempo is often stated relatively with words like *slow*, *medium* and *fast*. Try to develop a sense of tempo using these words because that's how you often talk about it. But beware: tempo is relative to the listener. What's *fast* to you may be *medium* to me. Still, try to develop a sense of what you consider slow, medium and fast. Then you can pretend to know something about music with lines like, "Gee, I like this tune. The uptempo beat is infectious and I couldn't stop tapping my foot." *Uptempo* means a fast tempo.

Here are my rough tempo ranges for slow, medium and fast. These ranges have evolved from partner dancing:

Slow – below 100 bpm
Medium – 100 bpm to 140 bpm
Fast – above 140 bpm

I find it helpful to add a "medium slow," which is about 100 to 110 bpm; and a "medium fast," which is about 125 to 140 bpm. Above 200 bpm I call *very* fast—or "way too fast to dance."

Occasionally, a song will have a tempo change but that's uncommon. "Stairway to Heaven" by Led Zeppelin is an example of a song with three tempos; the tempo increases as the song progresses. Occasionally, just the opening section of a piece of music, what's called the *introduction*, has a different tempo.

DANCING ALERT: Most dance teachers use slower tempos to teach because that makes it easier to learn to dance. But beware: sometimes a step pattern that you danced beautifully in class at, say, 105 bpm will fall apart at a social dance at, say, 125 bpm, because of the faster pace.

ARCANE INFO ALERT: To my chagrin, some styles of ballroom dancing count tempo in measures per minute. Counting in measures makes no sense. Don't do it!

In some genres of music the range of tempos is narrow, and in some genres the range is broad. Same with dance: some dances are danced in a narrow range of tempos, some in a broad range. Here are a few examples to give you a taste (*note:* not everyone agrees on tempo ranges so consider my numbers approximate).

House music, a type of electronic dance music (EDM), has a tempo range of 120 to 130 bpm, which is a popular tempo range in club dancing. *Downtempo,* also a type of EDM, has slower tempos, in the range of 90 to 120 bpm. *Salsa* has a tempo range of 160 to 220 bpm. *Cha-cha* has a range of 110 to 130 bpm. Both *waltz* and *swing* music span a broad range. *Rock and roll* also covers a full spectrum of tempos.

Sometimes tempo can help me identify the musical genre of a song. For example, I use it to help distinguish the different subgenres of Latin music. Salsa music is fast and cha-cha is medium tempo. So when I hear fast Latin music, I immediately rule out cha-cha and consider salsa.

The popularity of workout music has exploded in recent years. There are now many dedicated websites for workout music, with some giving you specific tempo ranges to suit various exercises. Most workout music falls in the range of 120 to 140 bpm. For warming up or for an easy workout, you'd go for less than 120 bpm. For high-intensity cardio, you'd go for a range of 140 to 160 bpm. (*Note:* these numbers are approximate.)

How to Calculate Tempo

(If my spiel that follows on calculating tempo is too tedious, I suggest you skip directly to the instructional video, **video 5.1,** then come back to this.)

If only there were tempo detection software that could magically tell you the bpm. Well, they exist, but I'm not convinced their accuracy is up to snuff. They seem to do a good job, but they make errors. I want 100 percent accuracy with tempo, so I prefer to do it myself, but if I needed to calculate the tempos for a 1,000-song library all at once, I'd probably use one. If anyone has a recommendation, I'm all ears.

Manually calculating tempo is easy to do, really. And once you know how, you can sometimes use the tempo to help you confirm that you found the beat. I'll explain how that works in a moment.

Before the internet, to calculate tempo you'd do something like count the number of beats you hear in 10 seconds, then multiply that number by six (10 seconds x 6 = 1 minute), which gave you beats per minute. It was not too accurate.

Nowadays, there are "tap tempo" websites and apps, which are superior and a cinch to use. You listen to a piece of music for the beat, then manually tap out the beat on a key on your keyboard or a button on the screen of your smartphone. The program simply displays how fast you're tapping in bpm. Voila.

What "tap tempo" won't do is magically tell you the tempo. You have to tap on time, so it's just a simple way to measure how fast you tap. If your dog tapped the key in dead silence, it would also display a number. If you tap the tempo incorrectly, you will get an incorrect bpm. So the hitch is that you need to be sure of the beat.

When I'm on my computer, I tap tempos using either **all8.com/tools/bpm** or **tempotap.com**. When I'm on my iPhone, I use the app **Tap/Tempo**. There are others out there that I've not looked at. These programs worked, and they weren't cluttered with other features, so I stopped looking. Just search the web for "tap tempo" and you'll find other choices.

Note that tapping tempo with a finger involves some coordination. It takes a little practice and focus to be accurate and consistent. So if tap tempo doesn't work for you, consider that the problem is coordination and not an inability to hear the beat. Practice and you'll get better.

Once you get good at tapping the beat, it should take less than 10 seconds to calculate the tempo using a tap tempo smartphone app or website. Really, if you have a good finger and can tap it steadily for a few seconds, it's that fast.

Before you look at the next video of tap tempo in action, I want to introduce another tempo tool, then I'll demonstrate them together. That tool is a bpm database, which is handy to know about because you can sometimes use it to confirm that you found the beat. A bpm database is a website for looking up the bpm of songs. Currently, I use **songbpm.com**.

To calculate tempo, check out **video 5.1**, "How to Calculate Music Tempo." Although this may not always work, the video also shows how to use a bpm database, along with a tap tempo app, to test yourself (albeit crudely) if you've found the beat. Here are the steps:

1. Count the sets of 8 to find the beat.

2. Calculate the tempo using a tap tempo website or app.

3. Go to songbpm.com. Enter the artist and title of the song. Wham, bam, you've got the tempo.

4. Compare it to your calculation. If you're right on, congrats.

From this point on I do some guessing:

• If you're within two or three beats, you're probably accurately counting the sets of 8. The discrepancy may be due to a slight inaccuracy in your tapping. When I'm off by a few beats, I tap again with a steadier finger, which, if anything, helps to train my coordination. Generally, if I'm within a beat or two, that's accurate enough for me, especially if it's a fast tempo.

• If you think your tapping is accurate and you're still off by a few beats to, say, 10 beats, consider the possibility that you're listening to a different recording of the song with a slightly different tempo. Sometimes you can see this in the songbpm.com results because it lists different versions of a song with slightly different tempos. For example, there could be two listings, a studio recording at 120 bpm and a live performance at 125 bpm.

• If you're way off, the first thing to do is see if your calculation is one-half of what the bpm database reports (e.g., you calculate 80 bpm, the database reports 160 bpm); or if it's the opposite, so your calculation is double what the database reports (e.g., you calculate 160 bpm, it reports 80 bpm). In this case, go back to the song and see if you can count "fast sets of 8" that are double your original speed, or "slow sets of 8" that are one-half your original speed, respectively. Tap the new tempo and see if it now matches the database. I'll give an example of this in a moment.

- If you're moderately off to way off (say, 15 beats or more) consider that you're inaccurately hearing the beat. Try again or move on to an easier song. Save the title for later so you can go back to it.

- If you're way off or get bad results with songbpm .com, there's also the possibility that there's something about the song (e.g., the song has tempo changes) or that the database is inaccurate. So you may get curve balls when using this database and it's best to keep your expectations low. I use it as a blunt tool and I try not to get hung up on one song if things are a little out of whack. Also, lesser-known songs will not be listed.

In video 5.1 I calculate the tempo for two versions of the song "Layla," both by Eric Clapton. The first recording, at

94 bpm, is Clapton doing an acoustic, unplugged version. The second is the original recording of the song, at 115 bpm, when Clapton was with Derek and the Dominos. How much does the decrease in tempo contribute to the new, mellow feeling of the song? That's hard to know, so the question is more to get you actively thinking about tempo.

I occasionally run into music with a challenging tempo. Typically, a hard song for me is when I can count both "slow sets of 8" and "fast sets of 8." Sometimes listening very closely will help me figure it out (listening for the natural pairing of beats, discussed in Chapter 3, can help). Sometimes thinking less and letting my foot intuitively tap it out will work. Sometimes plugging the song and artist into songbpm.com will help, but then again, sometimes songbpm.com is inaccurate. (I suspect that the tempo-detection software used by the database has trouble, just like my ear, with songs that have both slow sets of 8 and fast sets of 8.)

Here's the funny thing: I've run into songs that have two tempos listed at songbpm.com, the faster one being about twice the slower tempo. When I wrote the first draft of this chapter, the example I wanted to give was "Before He Cheats" by Carrie Underwood, which was listed at both 74 and 148 bpm. Note that multiplying 74 by two gives you 148. But today (in March 2017), as I do the final edit on this chapter, the slow tempo has been removed and songbpm.com only lists the faster tempo, 148 bpm. I can't find another example that I like of a song with two tempos listed, but we can still discuss "Before He Cheats." That's because there's another bpm database on the web, conveniently called **bpmdatabase.com**, which lists the tempo at 74 bpm. This shows you how, on occasion, it can be a challenge to confirm the correct tempo.

So which is the accurate tempo for "Before He Cheats"? I believe it's the slow sets of 8, so I believe songbpm.com is not accurate. I hear the natural pairing of beats, a faint "boom TICK" every two beats, which is at 74 bpm. That's my final answer.

Go to the website and watch **video 5.2**, "Before He Cheats" by Carrie Underwood. First, without counting, can you hear both slow sets of 8 and fast sets of 8? Then try to count the sets of 8 at the two different tempos. There's a link to a tap tempo website, if you want to tap out the two tempos. There are also links to songbpm.com and bpmdatabase.com so you can see the song listed at the two different tempos, although periodically the information on these websites gets updated so I don't know how they'll read when you get there.

TIP: Here's another way to find the tempo, but it doesn't always work. Search the web for the sheet music (just add the phrase "sheet music" to the name of the song), which sometimes gives you a *tempo marking* on the first page (usually, the first page is free so you won't have to buy the whole song). Sometimes, at the top of the page there will be a notation of a musical note (a quarter note), then an equal sign ("="), then a number, which is the bpm. It won't say "bpm" after the number so it seems a little mysterious, but that's the tempo.

$$\text{♩} = 120 \qquad \text{120 bpm}$$

There's one other thing I want to mention with regard to tempo. Sometimes a piece of music has a feeling or energy that's faster or slower than the actual tempo. For example, the music may have a fast energy but the tempo is slow. If you're trying to connect to the beat, don't be conflicted— the tempo is the tempo, which is beats per minute. It's not always the energy of the song.

"Kryptonite" by 3 Doors Down is an example of a higher-energy song with a slower tempo. The tempo is 99 bpm, which is slow, but the song sounds fast. Go to the website and watch **video 5.3**. Count the sets of 8 to find the beat, then tap the tempo.

Finally, once you get the tempo of a song in your music collection you can enter it into your music program on your computer. I use iTunes, and it seems like the way to enter it changes every few years so I won't go over it here. The easiest way to find the current method is to google something like "set bpm in iTunes 12." Note that I put the version number for iTunes (12), otherwise you may get results for older versions of iTunes.

Getting comfy with tempo isn't hard. Go ahead, give it a try and tap out a tempo or two.

Tell me what you listen to,
and I'll tell you who you are.

— Tiffanie DeBartolo,
author of *How to Kill a Rock Star*

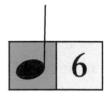

Phrasing

…every song contains audible clues that basically yell, "Hey, everyone, this is a new part!" These clues might include a new instrument that starts playing, a big crash, a drum fill or even just a significant change in the drum patterns. Electronic music loves to steadily add and subtract different parts every 32 counts, making it easy to recognize and work with those changes.

— Ean Golden, http://www.djtechtools.com/ 2009/01/26/phrasing-the-perfect-mix

…music can be abstract and there is often more than one correct answer to a phrasing question. You might get different teachers telling you to phrase differently. Just remember, you are dealing with the expression of ideas. Ideas change and are interpreted in different ways.

— Bradford Werner, http://www.thisis classicalguitar.com/phrasing-in-music

NOTE: Phrasing is hard! While sets of 8 are usually easy to identify once you get the hang of it, phrasing is not. Not only can the phrasing of a song be open to interpretation, but also with newer music there are more and more songs with weird or unidentifiable phrasing. I include this chapter because you need to be aware of phrasing, but don't get hung up on trying to identify the phrasing of a song. *Hearing the sets of 8 is the primary skill you need to learn.*

YOU'RE HANGING OUT WITH FRIENDS and listening to music. It's music nobody's heard before. A guy in the group starts getting into it. He bounces around and plays a little air guitar. His movements build in intensity. Then he punches the air with his fist precisely when the music hits a big accent. He's never heard this music before, so how'd he catch that accent with his fist?

One way to do it is with talent. For the rest of us, we can do it by becoming more musical. You'll learn more about that in the next chapter. But for starters, learning how to identify the bigger structure of music, called **phrasing**, is a good first step toward becoming more musical.

Guess what? You already know phrasing. All our talk of mini-phrases (sets of 8) and major phrases (four sets of 8) in Chapter 1 is phrasing. LINGO ALERT: Musicians, singers and dancers may use the word *phrasing* in somewhat different ways. When you hear the word, note the source and take it in context.

The first two songs from Chapter 1 are examples of *simple phrasing* ("Brother Louie" and "Gotta Do Some War

Work, Baby," which I count in video 1.5). Simple phrasing is music that's structured in four sets of 8. That is, four eight-beat *mini-phrases* come together to create a 32-beat *major phrase* of music.

While simple phrasing is common, it's not the only way that music is structured. Music can be phrased in many different and unusual ways. Compared to identifying the sets of 8, the phrasing can be elusive and difficult to identify. Phrasing can be complicated or confusing. Or it might even seem to not exist. But it's usually there. Even simple phrasing can be hard to identify because it can be soft or subtle. It's common to have to listen to a song more than once to be sure of the phrasing.

But here's the beauty of phrasing: usually, the structure of music repeats throughout a song. So if you identify the phrasing early on, you can predict where the rest of the song is going, even with unfamiliar music. *Not always, but often.*

For example, take the "punching the air" scenario presented in the opening paragraph of this chapter. If the music builds and hits with a big accent, that sequence will probably occur again (and maybe several times). So if you miss a big accent in the beginning of a song, you can be ready when it hits again. *That's one way you can know when to punch the air to a big accent even if you're listening to the song for the first time.* (You'll learn how to do it *spontaneously* in the back half of Chapter 7 in the exercise called "the spontaneous punch.")

Before we get into the details, listen to a few more songs with simple phrasing. Try to get a feel for how four sets of 8 come together to create a major phrase. Go to HearTheBeatFeelTheMusic.com and watch **video 6.1**, "Count Music–32-Beat Major Phrases."

Phrasing 101

Let's take a closer look at phrasing. I'll go through what to listen for, how to count a major phrase and how to notate the phrasing. This might be a little geeky, but I'll be gentle.

In Chapter 1, I talked about how a **mini-phrase** (also known as a *set of 8* in 4/4 time and a *set of 6* in 3/4 time) can have a theme or musical sense to it. But while the themes of mini-phrases have some integrity or completeness to them, they don't tell the whole story. A mini-phrase, like a sentence of words in a paragraph, only tells part of the story.

That's where the major phrase comes in. In the same way that a series of sentences come together to form a paragraph of words that tells the whole story, a series of mini-phrases come together to form a **major phrase** that tells the whole story. So the theme of a major phrase typically encompasses the smaller themes of the mini-phrases to create a larger theme, which is a *complete musical thought*.

For example, a common theme in music is what I call *setup and resolution*, which you first learned about in Chapter 1. "Brother Louie" and "Gotta Do Some War Work, Baby" are both good examples of setup and resolution (video 1.5). In all of the major phrases in both of these songs a theme builds in the first three sets of 8 that then gets resolved in the fourth set of 8.

But there's a catch with major phrases: the number of mini-phrases in a major phrase can vary. So even though four sets of 8 is very common, you'll be up against other arrangements as well. For example, six sets of 8, which would be a 48-beat major phrase, is common. It's considered standard phrasing for blues music (and it's sometimes used in other musical genres). LINGO ALERT: Musicians call music in 48-beat major phrases "12-bar blues," a *bar* being slang for a *measure* (12 bars × 4 beats/bar = 48 beats).

There's another catch, which is called "mixed phrasing," and this is where things get really tricky. The number of mini-phrases in the major phrases can vary throughout a song. So, for example, the first major phrase could be four sets of 8 and the next one could be five sets of 8. Or maybe you get one that's only three sets of 8. Sometimes you get a 16-beat phrase (two sets of 8) and you wonder, does it stand on its own as a 16-beat phrase or "bridge"? Or does it belong to the major phrase before it? Don't worry about it. You may never know the answer. Just roll with it. If you're choreographing, do your own interpretation.

Also, there's "irregular phrasing," which is when a song has extra beats. It can be any number of beats but usually an even number. For example, you might get two or four beats placed between major phrases.

But don't sweat. Like I said earlier, patterns that you hear in the beginning of a song usually repeat. So after you hear the first part of the song and can figure out the phrasing, you should have a good idea of how the rest will go. *Again, it doesn't always work out that way, but it often works.*

We'll get to more videos of counting the phrasing in a moment. First, here are the steps to identify the phrasing. These steps are not set in stone, they're just to get you going:

1. Count the sets of 8 to connect to the beat.

2. As you count sets of 8, listen for the beginning of a major phrase. TIP: Listen for the resolution or conclusion of a major phrase, which will signal that a new major phrase is about to start. For example, the transition between the chorus and verse is often easy to hear.

3. When a new major phrase begins, keep counting the sets of 8, but now keep track of the sets of 8 as they go by. Count the sets of 8 of a 32-beat major phrase like this (note that the **count 1s** escalate with each new set of 8):

   1 2 3 4   5 6 7 8
   2 2 3 4   5 6 7 8
   3 2 3 4   5 6 7 8
   4 2 3 4   5 6 7 8

4. When a new major phrase starts again, start the count over to keep track of the sets of 8 in the new

major phrase (i.e., go back to counting the number "1" on the first beat of the new major phrase). Two 32-beat major phrases would be counted like this:

1 2 3 4   5 6 7 8 – *first* major phrase
2 2 3 4   5 6 7 8
3 2 3 4   5 6 7 8
4 2 3 4   5 6 7 8

1 2 3 4   5 6 7 8 – *second* major phrase
2 2 3 4   5 6 7 8
3 2 3 4   5 6 7 8
4 2 3 4   5 6 7 8

5. If you like, keep track of the major phrases by creating a *musical skeleton*, explained in a moment.

6. You won't know if you're counting correctly until you count a few major phrases to see if it works out. It'll be trial and error, so you just have to jump in and start counting. There's often guesswork involved.

7. If you stumble—if the count doesn't seem to be correct—stop and start over. For example, you might hear a big transition when you weren't expecting it. Was that the beginning of a new major phrase? Perhaps, so start over counting from there and see if that works.

8. At first, practice with easy music. You know the routine: you need to hear the phrasing in the easy stuff before you hear it in the harder stuff.

To make practicing easier, I wish I could direct you to a genre of easy music that's always in 32-beat major phrases. But the best I can do is suggest music that has mostly simple phrasing. Two genres to try are big band swing music (jazz) and electronic dance music (EDM). Also, most partner dancing music and dance fitness music (aerobics, Zumba, etc.) should be easy music. Most of that music has simple phrasing (four sets of 8) because that's a quality that makes it good for dancing and dance fitness.

Lets look at more phrasing in action. Go to the website and watch the **video series 6.2**, "Count Music–32-Beat Phrasing." All the songs will be simple phrasing (I count just part of each song; if the simple phrasing doesn't extend to the entire song, the section I count will be 32-beat phrases).

DANCING ALERT: As a dancer, my ear wants to hear 32-beat phrases because those are the easiest to dance to. So if the phrasing is subtle or open to interpretation, I will interpret it in 32-beat major phrases.

As you listen to music throughout your day, you're likely to hear a variety of phrasing. If you try to count your everyday music, you're going to bump into songs where the major phrasing is hard to identify or open to interpretation. And even if you think you know the correct phrasing, you may not be sure and there is no way to check. That's right, there's no easy way to confirm the phrasing. Don't get hung up on it. If you listen to a song three or four times and still don't get it, it's best to move on to the next song.

Musical Skeletons

Sometimes you get a song that you want to work on, a song that you want to pull apart and really figure out. Here's what you do.

First, capture the name of the song so you can listen to it over and over. Try music recognition apps like SoundHound and Shazam.

Then, boy oh boy, have I got a treat for you: *musical skeletons*. They're a great way to help you identify and document the phrasing. I explain them below but you already got a taste of them in **video 2.4**. Go back and watch a bit of that video. Note that my left hand on the left side of the video is pointing at the musical skeleton.

A **musical skeleton** is just a notation, essentially a map, of how the mini-phrases (sets of 8) are grouped in a song. If you're choreographing a routine to a song, do a musical skeleton. They're darn simple. (Credit to Swing Dance Hall of Famer Skippy Blair for musical skeletons.) Here's how they work:

- You note a set of 8 with the numeral "8" like this: 8. So a major phrase composed of four sets of 8 gets noted like this: 8888.

- A song with a major phrase composed of six sets of 8 gets noted like this: 888888.

- For a waltz, you note a set of 6 with the numeral "6" like this: 6. So a major phrase composed of four sets of 6 gets noted like this: 6666.

- If you get a more complicated song with a phrase that's only, say, four beats, you note it like this: 4. For example, "Yesterday" by the Beatles has some major phrases made up of three sets of 8 followed by one set of 4. That gets noted like this: 8884. (*Note:* As I go to press, YouTube blocked the video I made of "Yesterday," but you can find the song on your own and try counting.)

- Start each new major phrase on a new line like this:
  8888 – first major phrase (32 beats)
  8888 – second major phrase (32 beats)
  8888
  etc.

- Feel free to jot notes on the skeleton describing whatever you want. For example, the word "intro" on the first line of the skeleton that follows is a descriptive note.

- I haven't talked much about *intros*, but typically a song has an *introduction*, which sounds a little different—occasionally, an intro is really weird—and leads you into the first major phrase. The intro can be any length, and I've noted the intro on the skeleton that follows as two sets of 8.

That's about it, really. Below is a generic musical skeleton for a song that has all simple phrasing, except for the

16-beat intro (I'm just showing the beginning of the song as the structure repeats):

```
88 – intro
8888
8888
8888
8888
etc.
```

In **video 6.3**, "Count Music–48-Beat Phrasing," I count a few songs structured in 48-beat phrases using a musical skeleton. Here's a generic musical skeleton for a song that has all 48-beat major phrases with a 32-beat intro:

```
8888 – intro
888888
888888
888888
888888
etc.
```

I don't want to dwell on hard music, but I'd like to give a few examples of songs that are a little bit harder because it'll prepare you for what you might encounter. I think anything that departs from 32-beat major phrases is usually another level of difficulty.

Go to the website and watch **video 6.4**, "Count Music–Complicated Phrasing." These songs are examples of mixed phrasing and irregular phrasing. Even though they're harder songs, I hope they're easy enough for you to quickly hear what's going on. For me, a hard song would be something I listen to four or five times and I still don't know what's going on. I regularly encounter songs that are too hard or ambiguous and I give up.

Alrighty then, that's a wrap on phrasing. If you're having trouble with it, don't fret, it'll make more sense over time. *Remember, newbies should focus on hearing sets of 8, which is the primary skill you need to know.* And take comfort in knowing that even when you struggle to hear the sets of 8 and the phrasing, you're training your ear because you're actively listening to music.

NOTES

Somebody just gave me a shower radio.
Thanks a lot. Do you really want music
in the shower? I guess there's no better
place to dance than a slick surface
next to a glass door.

— JERRY SEINFELD

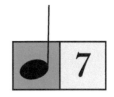

Move to Music

NOTE: The six excerpts below are on the biology of the human connection to music. They might be a little geeky, so you can skip them for now (not to worry, I summarize them in the first paragraph below the six excerpts). Also, while this chapter is more geared to dance and simply listening to music for enjoyment, quotes 4 and 5 that follow speak directly to the benefit of music when exercising.

> 1) *One of the most curious effects of music is that it compels us to move in synchrony with its beat. This behavior, also referred to as entrainment, includes spontaneous or deliberate finger and foot tapping, head nodding, and body swaying. The most striking of these phenomena is dancing: a human universal typically involving whole-body movements. Dancing rests on humans' unique ability to tightly couple auditory-motor circuits.*
> — Marcel Zentner and Tuomas Eerola
> "Rhythmic Engagement with Music in Infancy"

http://www.ncbi.nlm.nih.gov/pmc/articles/PMC2851927
(U.S. National Library of Medicine,
National Institutes of Health)

2) *The ability to follow a beat is called beat induction. Neither chimpanzees nor bonobos— our closest primate relatives—are capable of beat induction, which is considered both a uniquely human trait and a cognitive building block of music....*

"We hear music, we clap along. Music becomes faster or slower, and we can dance to it," said Honing [Henkjan Honing of the University of Amsterdam's Music Cognition Group], *lead author of the study, published Monday in the Proceedings of the National Academy of Sciences* ["Newborn Infants Detect the Beat in Music" Vol. 106, No. 4, Jan. 26, 2009].

— Brandon Keim
"Baby Got Beat: Music May Be Inborn"
http://www.wired.com/2009/01/babybeats

3) [Neuroscientist Valorie Salimpoor of the Rotman Research Institute in Toronto, Canada, and Robert Zatorre at McGill University's Montreal Neurological Institute] *...showed that listeners' dopamine levels in pleasure centers surged during key passages of favorite music, but also just a moment before—as if the brain was anticipating the crescendo to come.*

...Our brains are well-suited to using patterns, such as the structure of music, to predict the future. "We're constantly making predictions, even if we don't know the music," Salimpoor says. "We're still predicting how it should unfold."

These predictions are based on past musical experience, so classical fans will have different expectations than punk devotees. But when the music turns out better than the brain expected, the nucleus accumbens fires off with delight.
— Paul Gabrielsen
"Why Your Brain Loves That New Song"
http://news.sciencemag.org/2013/04/
why-your-brain-loves-new-song

4) *In fact, it's music's dual ability to distract attention (a psychological effect) while simultaneously goosing the heart and the muscles (physiological impacts) that makes it so effective during everyday exercise. Multiple experiments have found that music increases a person's subjective sense of motivation during a workout, and also concretely affects his or her performance.*

[Later in the article, Nina Kraus, a professor of neurobiology at Northwestern University in Illinois, who studies the effects of music on the nervous system, is quoted.] *"Humans and songbirds"* are the only creatures *"that automatically feel the beat"* of a song, she said. The human heart wants to synchronize to music, the legs want to swing, *metronomically, to a beat. So the next time you go for a moderate run or bike ride, first increase the tempo of some insidiously catchy Lady Gaga downloads (or Justin Bieber or Katy Perry or whatever reflects the current popular taste in your household), and load them on your iPod. "Our bodies," Dr. Kraus concluded, "are made to be moved by music and move to it."*

— Gretchen Reynolds
"Phys Ed: Does Music Make You Exercise Harder?"
http://well.blogs.nytimes.com/2010/08/25/
phys-ed-does-music-make-you-exercise-harder/?_r=0

5) *In the last 10 years the body of research on workout music has swelled considerably, helping psychologists refine their ideas about why exercise and music are such an effective pairing for so many people as well as how music changes the body and mind during physical exertion. Music distracts people from pain and fatigue, elevates mood, increases endurance, reduces perceived effort and may even promote metabolic efficiency. When listening to music, people run farther, bike longer and swim faster than usual—often without realizing it. In a 2012 review of the research, Costas Karageorghis of Brunel University in London, one of the world's leading experts on the psychology of exercise music, wrote that one could think of music as "a type of legal performance-enhancing drug."*

[Later in the article, cognitive neuroscientist Jessica Grahn of Western University's Brain and

Mind Institute in Ontario, Canada, is quoted.]
"We have also known for decades that there are direct connections from auditory neurons to motor neurons," explains Grahn, who enjoys working out to cheesy techno-music. *"When you hear a loud noise, you jump before you have even processed what it is. That's a reflex circuit, and it turns out that it can also be active for non-startling sounds, such as music."*

— Ferris Jabr
"Let's Get Physical: The Psychology of
Effective Workout Music"
http://www.scientificamerican.com/article/
psychology-workout-music

6) *Okay, but why? Why should a collection of sounds cause the brain to reward itself? That remains a bit of a mystery, but a favorite theory, proposed almost 60 years ago, posits that it's about fulfilled expectations. Put simply, music sets up patterns that causes us to predict what will come next and when we're right, we get a reward. Some have suggested this has its roots in primitive times when guessing wrong about animal sounds was a matter of life or death. What was needed was a quick emotional response to save our skin, rather than taking the time to think things through.*

— Randy Rieland
"Eight New Things We've Learned About Music"
http://www.smithsonianmag.com/innovation/
eight-new-things-weve-learned-about-music-40481109

THERE ARE REAL-LIFE, honest-to-God scientists who study the biological and psychological effects of music on humans. It's a field called biomusicology. According to biomusicology (from the previous excerpts), humans have a natural ability to connect to music:

- Music naturally makes us want to move.

- Once we're moving, our bodies will synchronize to the music, which is called *entrainment*.

- Music can produce a number of psychological and physical effects, which can lead to a better athletic performance and more enjoyment of the music.

- The human brain is good with pattern recognition, so we have some ability to predict what's coming next in the music, which adds to our listening pleasure.

The goal of this book has been to unlock and deepen your natural connection to music. You've learned how to count sets of 8 because it's the first step in becoming rhythmic. You've learned how to identify the phrasing and predict where the music is going because that's an important step toward better musicality. You've even started moving to music through clapping and snapping your fingers. Let's finish with a couple more things to help you move to music.

The first thing, tapping your foot, is drop-dead simple. The second thing, "the spontaneous punch," is much harder. Yup, we're going to circle back to the scenario I set up in the Introduction and in Chapter 6: that is, how to listen to a song for the first time and be able to predict a big accent and punch the air. I'm going to deliver on that punch—and take it to the next level.

Tap Your Foot

If you don't already, start tapping your foot to music.

I know what you're thinking: *Foot-tapping? Really? It's a throwaway move. Irrelevant.*

Not really. Many people naturally tap. It's one of the first indications that you're becoming *entrained* by the music. Your body wants to move and tapping is the minimal, entry-level move. It's easy, familiar and comfortable. It's pleasurable, in a calming and meditative way. It's a socially accepted way of "getting into the music" without the self-consciousness of dancing. It can even be done privately because you can tap your big toe inside your shoe and nobody will know.

And tapping can also look cool. Rock stars tap their feet.

Imagine that you're watching a dance floor, like at a wedding reception or at a club. You could stand there all stiff with your arms folded. Or you could drop your arms, relax, crack a smile and gently tap your foot. Much cooler. If you're hoping someone will ask you to dance, this is a good look (TIP: stand at the edge of the dance floor).

Imagine you're at a concert. You could sit there like an icicle, all analytical and in your head. Or you could take a deep breath, release the scrunch from your shoulders and tap your toe. Get into the groove. I bet you'll enjoy the music more.

I know what you're thinking: *Tap schmap. Tapping seems dumb. I'm cool already. Why should I care about tapping?*

Here's something that works for me, and maybe it'll work for you. I use my foot-tapping as another clue to help me find the beat and connect to the music. Over the years my foot-tapping accuracy—the ability to tap on the beat—has improved. Now when I naturally tap, I'm virtually always on the beat. Based on the principal of *entrainment* (from the first quote at the start of this chapter), this makes sense. Now when I'm up against a hard song, I'll let my foot naturally tap. This gives me intuitive feedback, which helps me confirm that I'm on the beat. I use it like a gauge to sniff out the beat.

Tapping is an easy way to connect to music. It's fun to tap with confidence. Play with it.

Got Musicality?

musicality: The ability to hear specific changes in the music that warrant interpretation. The ability to feel mood changes in the music and interpret that change with body movement that accentuates the feeling in the music.

— Skippy Blair
Skippy Blair's Dance Terminology Dictionary, 5th edition

Musicality in dance then might be considered a measure or degree to which a dancer is receptive and creative in his translation or rendering of music through movement.

— Nichelle Suzanne
http://www.danceadvantage.net/musicality-in-dance

The word *musicality* is sometimes used, incorrectly, to mean an ability to hear the beat. Musicality is much deeper than that. It has to do with hearing something in the music, like an accent or a riff or a mood, and artistically interpreting that musical element with a movement of the body. It's even deeper than that because true musicality may involve talent, but I'm going to leave that discussion for another day.

Can anybody improve their musicality? I don't know. I think most people can become more "musical" if they work at it. My goal in the rest of this chapter is to help you become more musical by working on feeling the music and moving spontaneously.

The best way to understand what I want to help you with is to see it in action. Check out this couple dancing. See how their dancing artistically matches what's going on in the music. Go to HearTheBeatFeelTheMusic.com and watch **video 7.1**, "Musicality in West Coast Swing." (If you read the YouTube comments, you'll see this dance was not choreographed. But I presume both dancers were familiar with the song and had danced together before.)

Moving spontaneously to music is a two-step process. The first step is "musical receptivity," which is perceiving or recognizing an element in music that's worthy of interpretation (like an accent, riff or mood change). I believe this is a skill or "muscle" you can exercise. I think this is the harder part and we're going to work on it in a moment with the punching exercise.

The second step is to creatively interpret the musical element through body movement and dance. We're not going to work on this, but I'll break it down now in a practical way so that you can learn it on your own:

- *You need to have a repertoire of "moves" to perform* (or be able to improvise a new move). To do this, you can learn moves off YouTube or take dance classes.

- *You need technique to make those moves look good.* This could be hard to learn on your own. You'll probably need someone who can explain the technique behind body movement. Then you have to practice, a lot. Dance classes are a place to learn this, but they don't always go into the technique of movement. Check out the teacher before you go.

- *You need an artistic sense to choose a move to fit or express an element in the music.* This is a tough one. If you don't have an artistic eye, I think you have to watch a lot of great dancers to develop your eye. And you have to experiment to develop your personal style. Even if you're not much of an artist, you can have fun with your own style and still gain the admiration of others. *You have to learn to make the dance your own.*

In the exercise that follows, you're just going to punch the air. The punch is the "move." So, in this exercise, you won't work on technique or creativity because a punch requires none of that. Instead, you're going to work on "receiving" the music by practicing a spontaneous punch.

What do I mean by *spontaneous*?

In dance, I like to distinguish between two types of movement: sometimes the movement is planned; and sometimes it's unplanned or spontaneous.

Movement is planned when you listen to a song over and over and choreograph a dance routine. Virtually everything you see on the stage, on TV and in the movies is planned. In a similar way, when you're dancing to a song you've heard many times before, what you do could be planned (or partially planned) because you know what's coming in the music. In all of these situations you've had many chances to hear or receive the music.

Movement can also be planned to unfamiliar music. You were introduced to that concept in Chapter 6 when I revealed how to punch the air to a big accent. You learned that the structure of a song usually repeats. So even if you miss a musical element in the beginning of a song, like a big accent, it usually repeats. In that sense, even though the first half of the song is unfamiliar, the second half of the song is somewhat familiar, which lets you respond to a big accent in a planned way. Essentially, you're given a second chance to receive the music.

But what if you could listen to an unfamiliar song and magically punch the air to the first big accent, even though you had no clue it was coming? Holy cow, that's spontaneous!

Spontaneity is rare to see in TV and film. It's more common in casual situations, like on a social dance floor or a street corner. Or, say, in your kitchen, where you're cooking dinner when nobody's watching and hopping around to a random tune. In these situations you have but one chance to receive music that's unfamiliar.

To be spontaneous you need the ability to react or "catch" something in the music. This is a thoughtless action. That's our path at the moment: "catching" stuff in music, which we'll express through a punch. Eventually, as you get better, what comes out of you—the "move"—may not be known by you or planned in advance. What comes out of you may not be what you'd expect and it may be something you've never done before. No kidding, it's like magic.

On to the punch!

The Spontaneous Punch

You're going to punch the air to a *break* in the music. A **break** is when the music builds, hits an accent and then seems to stop: most or all of the instruments and vocals cut out for a few seconds. Breaks are one of the easiest elements in music to hear, which makes them a good place to start.

This exercise is similar to an old concept in dance called "hitting the breaks." Hitting a break is acknowledging the dramatic change in the music (the break) with a dramatic dance move. At a basic level of dance you could freeze your body or strike a pose, which are moves that would artistically fit the silence you hear during a break. At a more advanced level, you could do something like a syncopation with your footwork or a styling move, like a body roll. With a partner you could do a dramatic move like a dip. Here's what I want you to do:

- When the music breaks, either punch or do something creative (suggestions follow). Breaks usually occur toward the end of a major phrase. Listen to a song and punch the air on the accented beat, which starts the break—usually a **count 1**, sometimes a **count 5**.

- Here's the challenge: *the first one or two times through each song, do not count.* Listen to the songs without counting the sets of 8. So the point of this exercise is to feel the music build up to the break and to predict, spontaneously, without counting, when the break will hit. This is also an exercise in getting a feel for the phrasing and structure.

- Then count the sets of 8 to see on which count the break starts. (You can also try to count the major phrases as if you were going to create a musical skeleton, but a lot of the phrasing is difficult so don't get hung up on this.)

- Your punch doesn't have to be pretty. A punch doesn't require any technique, so really you're off the hook. Heck, I don't care, you can do it lying down on a couch. A punch is hard to mess up.

- There's one artistic aspect of a punch you can control: the strength of your punch. If it's a big accent in the music, do a big punch; if it's a small accent, do a small punch. So, in addition to predicting the arrival of the accent, try to predict how hard the accent will hit.

- To add some creativity, instead of doing a punch, you could try other simple moves, like splaying your hands (extend your fingers wide open, like the styling move called "jazz hands," which you can google). Or you could simply point a finger, do a head flick, freeze your body, strike a pose—or why not just improvise and let anything come out? Try to surprise yourself. If you get serious about beefing up your repertoire of moves, poke around YouTube with search phrases like dance moves, dance club moves, hip-hop moves, jazz moves, jazz isolations, dance styling, etc. You could take a hip-hop class, too.

- *This is critical:* If you mistakenly punch an accent that isn't there, practice diffusing your punch. After you start the punch, let the energy rapidly drain from your fist and arm. Really, just let the energy vanish. Puff! It works. Recovering from mistakes is an important skill you need to learn. TIP: There's no reason to be self-conscious about making mistakes because mistakes always seem bigger to you than to an audience. Often an audience won't even see a mistake. ANOTHER TIP: There's on old saying in dance that goes something like, "There are no mistakes, only syncopations." So practice turning a mistake into a new move. AND ANOTHER TIP: There's another reason not to be self-conscious. *What people see can affect what they hear.* So, for example, if you deliver a *big* punch to a *tiny* accent, an audience may actually hear a bigger accent. That may not be a bad thing and it may even look good. So what you think is a mistake, the audience thinks is just another cool move.

Go to the website and watch **video series 7.2**, "Hitting the Breaks with a Spontaneous Punch." It's just music videos of songs that have breaks. Some of the songs have many breaks, some have only a couple. But all the songs should have at least two breaks. The hit on some breaks is strong and on some it's weak. Some of the breaks are four beats long, some are eight beats long.

Note that when you listen to each song for the first time the music will be unfamiliar. But obviously, after you've heard a song a couple of times and know what's coming, the music will be familiar. At that point your movement becomes more planned and less spontaneous. So these songs are to get you started. The real practice will be to actively listen for things to react to in your everyday music.

But if you listen for breaks in your everyday music, you may not hear that many or any at all. I don't know how common breaks are in the music of today, but my guess is that they're not common. I find them more commonly in blues, big band swing and oldies music from the 1960s. Listen to an oldies station and you should hear breaks.

Here's what to listen for in your everyday music. There are many strong accents in music that aren't associated with a break but are still worthy of a punch. As you know, it's common for a **count 1** to have an accent. You also know that it's common for the **count 1** of a new major phrase to have an even stronger accent. Try punching there, the **count 1** of a new major phrase. Granted, these may not always be loud accents, so simply adjust the size and intensity of your punch to match the accent. Got it? Do it!

DANCE TIP: Here's something to explore on YouTube. Some partner dancing competitions have a division called

"Jack and Jill," which is when your dance partner and the music are not known in advance. There's no planned choreography, and in that sense it's similar to a social dance floor. Even though one or both dancers may know the song, Jack and Jill competitions often have a good degree of spontaneity. Just search for Jack and Jill dance competitions.

For me, the hard part in achieving spontaneous movement to music was getting into the mindset and habit of consciously listening for things to react to. That is, I had to remember to do it. Then, after that, I had to train long enough until it became an unconscious action so I didn't have to think about it. Today, the intuitive side of my brain, my subconscious, is always listening to music in this deeper way. It's effortless.

Nowadays, it feels as if the music "pulls" stuff (moves) out of me. I like that word "pull" because it means I don't push or force the moves out. The music makes me do it. Granted, my moves are not always pretty because I'm not a highly trained dancer. But I'm pursuing one of the goals of better musicality: I'm making the dance my own.

> There will always be somebody who dances better than I do. And there will always be someone who dances much, much worse than I do. Confidence comes from "owning" what you do.
> — Skippy Blair, dance educator

Speaking of owning what you do, take a look at **video 7.3**, which is Pharrell Williams's "Happy." This is the four-minute official video for the song "Happy," which was pulled from 24 hours of shooting people on the street. It's a lot of everyday folks dancing their own thing. It's raw footage of dancing because each dancer got filmed in only one take.

DANCE TIP: This works for me, and I hope it works for you. When I dance, both my conscious mind and subconscious mind are constantly guessing what the music will do next. In a typical evening of dance, I make many mistakes in my guessing: that is, I *inaccurately* catch and react to things in the music that aren't there. No biggie, because I cover the mistakes (I let them diffuse so they don't look out of place). But I do catch a few spot on, which feels great. And that's what people see. People either don't see the misses or they forget them. So my advice is the same advice you'd get from any self-improvement book: *take chances and don't be afraid to fail.* These self-improvement books will then point out that this was the successful strategy used by Babe Ruth in 1923. In that year he not only broke the record for the most home runs, but he also broke the record for striking out.

Final Words: My Promise to You

I'm a guy who had zero musicality; actually, sub-zero. Improving my spontaneous movement to music in partner dancing has been incomprehensibly hard. I started by asking dancers who had great musicality how they did it. They said to listen to the music and react; listen hard and just do it. That didn't seem like much of a game plan. What I wanted was for them to reveal the secret to musicality, but it doesn't exist. I concluded that they all had talent, which I didn't have. I figured I'd never get it. I went through years of frustration.

But I came to realize that those talented dancers were correct. You have to work at it, and if you don't have talent, you have to work really, really hard. Eventually, for me "hitting the breaks" (from the punching exercise) became my gateway to improving my spontaneous movement because breaks in music are easy to hear.

In the beginning, hitting a break was hard even to familiar music (because I was distracted by other things like staying on the beat, leading my follower, choreographing the next move in my head, keeping my cool). Eventually, I could do it, but I'd be late by a beat or two. Finally, I could hit the breaks on time, even to unfamiliar music. After that, I began to loosen up, gain confidence and catch smaller things in the music. Mind you, my musicality is still not on anyone's radar screen, but I've become more musical.

And that's my promise to you. I don't care if you think you have no connection to music, no ability to hear the beat and no musicality. You probably have some ability with music, and if you put in the time and train, even if you don't become great, you will get better.

ONE MORE THING: Please give this book an honest review on Amazon because I need reviews. (If you're about to give it a 1-star review because YouTube blocked a video, please email me first at jim@ihatetodance.com)

ANSWER TO POP QUIZ IN CHAPTER 2: count 7
ANSWER TO POP QUIZ IN CHAPTER 3: at the 40 second mark

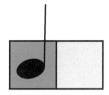

Meet the Author

JAMES JOSEPH first cracked the code to music and dance in his 2010 book *Every Man's Survival Guide to Ballroom Dancing.* He is a GSDTA certified dance instructor and has trained for more than 20 years under Swing Dance Hall of Fame member Skippy Blair. His other books include *Read Your Way to the Top, The Kreplachness Monster* and *Working Wonders: 60 Quick Break Techniques to Beat Burnout, Boost Productivity and Revive Your Work Day.*

Purchase Books

The two books below are available for purchase at online retailers, both in print and ebook. For more information:

Hear the Beat, Feel the Music
HearTheBeatFeelTheMusic.com

Every Man's Survival Guide to Ballroom Dancing
iHateToDance.com

Made in United States
Troutdale, OR
07/17/2023

11329980R00066